Jo Stepaniak, M
Vesanto Melina,
and Dina Aronson, MS, RD

Food Allergies

Health and Healing

books
Alive

Summertown
Tennessee

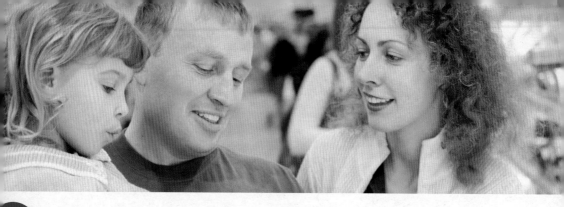

CONTENTS

Food Allergies

Recipes

Note: Conversions in this book (from imperial to metric) are not exact. They have been rounded to the nearest measurement for convenience. Exact measurements are given in imperial. The recipes in this book are by no means to be taken as therapeutic. They simply promote the philosophy of both the authors and Books Alive in relation to whole foods, health, and nutrition, while incorporating the practical advice given by the authors in the first section of the book.

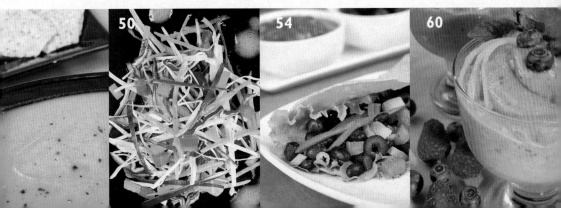

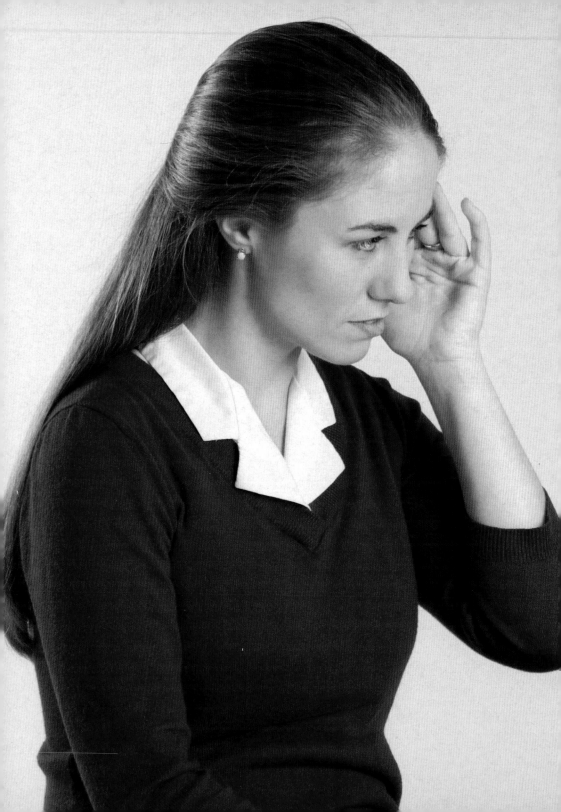

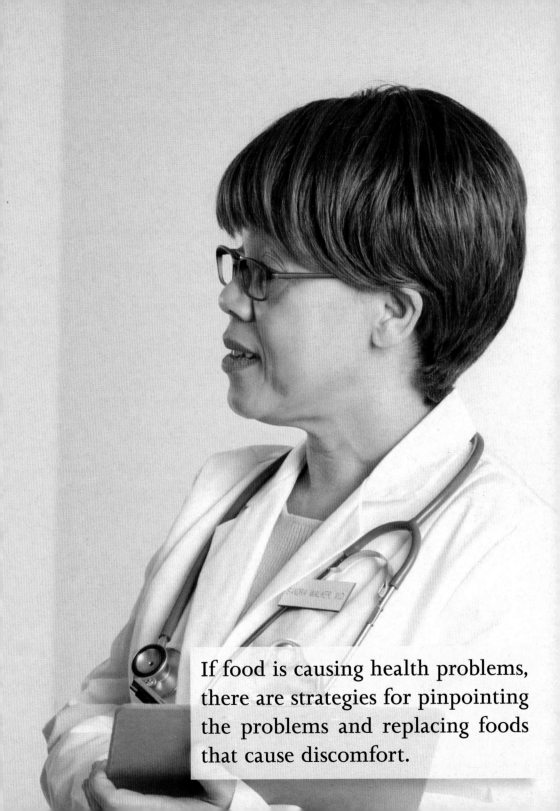

If food is causing health problems, there are strategies for pinpointing the problems and replacing foods that cause discomfort.

Introduction . . . .

During the course of our lifetimes, each of us will eat an estimated two to three tons of food. When food allergies arise, however, our intake may drop considerably, and our lives may be disrupted in many un-expected and challenging ways. Longtime favorite foods are banned from our homes. Familiar choices on restaurant menus are now off limits. And the easy ways in which we put meals together in the past are suddenly fraught with hurdles.

Fortunately, it is possible to enjoy an extensive and varied diet even when you have food allergies. In fact, with a little know-how, being well nourished becomes simple. Instead of viewing with despair a list of for-bidden foods, you can plan flavorful and appealing meals for the day. Your food allergies may even have beneficial side effects by shepherding you to a path of excellent health, a diet of nourishing whole foods, and a lifestyle that helps you avoid problematic situations or manage them gracefully.

What Are Food Allergies? . . . .

Reactions to food can be experienced in many different parts of your body and range from mild irritation to life-threatening anaphylactic responses. Food allergy is the reaction of the body's immune system to a food or food ingredient that it recognizes as "foreign." It is different from a food intolerance, which is an adverse reaction to a food, food ingredient, or additive that does not involve the immune system. A food intolerance typically involves the digestive system. The term "food sensitivity" includes both allergy and intolerance.

True food allergy, also known as food hypersensitivity, is actually a case of mistaken identity. Our symptoms are inappropriate (and often very uncomfortable) responses by the immune system to an otherwise harmless substance in food, typically a protein. If our immune system failed to respond as it does, that food would not pose a threat to us.

Food Allergy: Defense at Our Own Expense

The actions of the immune system against food allergens have many similarities to its actions against foreign bacteria or viruses. In both cir-cumstances the reactions follow this sequence:

1. Recognize the invader (in this case, a food fragment or molecule called an allergen).
2. Classify the invader as dangerous.
3. Prepare a tailor-made defense.
4. Destroy the invader by unleashing destructive chemicals.

The first time a food allergen, which is typically a protein, enters the body, it generally does not trigger an allergic reaction; however, the body becomes sensitized. During sensitization, the immune system is alerted to the presence of the allergen, determines that this substance poses a threat, and prepares its defense. The next time the allergen enters the body, the immune system is ready to launch its counter-attack. A complex series of events occurs, with each successive stage dependent upon the preceding stage.

Unlike foreign bacteria and viruses, food components do not typically cause disease and do not warrant this massive defense. Nonetheless, symptoms occur in those of us who experience food allergies. The immune system reacts to food proteins (allergens) by producing antibodies. These in turn cause mast cells and similar immune-system cells to release chemicals, causing inflammation. As in the protective response against potential disease, our tissues heat up. Access routes (blood vessels) widen to allow more chemicals to come to the defense. The body quickly produces more cells to join the defensive army. Body tissues may become red, swollen, and warm with the increased flow of blood and body fluids. Symptoms will differ depending on which part of the body is the site of the action: the skin, head, muscles around the lungs, mucous membranes in the nose or digestive tract, or other regions, as shown in the table on page 9. The weapons of defense hurt the body's own cells and result in mild to severe symptoms on the skin or in the respiratory, nervous, or digestive system.

OUR ARSENAL OF CHEMICAL WEAPONS

The inflammatory mediators that we release include histamine, prostaglandins, leukotrienes, and bradykinins, each with specific effects. Enzymes that may cause tissue damage are also released. Histamine is a powerful mediator that can do the following:

- cause blood vessels to widen
- allow fluids and proteins that are normally contained by blood vessels to leak through
- increase the secretion of mucus by mucous membranes
- cause muscles (such as those around the lungs) to contract
- stimulate nerves, creating an itch

Histamine can be created and released by mast cells in many parts of the body. Exactly what we experience depends on the area in which the histamine is acting.

Prostaglandins and leukotrienes (hormonelike chemicals made from fatty acids) and bradykinins (short chains of amino acids that affect blood pressure) can do the following:

- increase the dilation of blood vessels
- increase the secretion of mucus by mucous membranes
- cause constriction of muscles around the lungs
- control pain, swelling, and muscle contraction
- move cells containing inflammatory mediators from one place to another
- act on the nervous system and gastrointestinal tract

Symptoms of Food Allergies . . . .

Adverse reactions to foods can appear in various target areas of the body, as shown in the table on page 9. A reaction may appear in one location for one individual, whereas another person may have an entirely different experience. For many people the skin is particularly vulnerable to attack. Patches near the mouth or on another part of the face swell, redden, break out in hives, and itch, or eczema may develop on the hands and other parts of the body. For others, the nose becomes stuffy and runny or the lungs go into spasm. Some people develop mild or severe headaches. A common target area is the digestive tract, which can react to allergens from one end to the other. Many people show symptoms in more than one of these areas.

Severity of Symptoms

Symptoms range from mild irritation to severe responses involving the whole body. For some individuals, various influences can affect the severity of reactions. If more than one type of allergen is encountered at once, increased amounts of inflammatory chemicals may be released, heightening the response. Inflammation in the digestive system caused by infection, for example, can make it easier for allergens to get into the body, increasing the effects. Alcohol, when consumed at the same time as an allergen, can result in greater absorption of an allergen.

Although exercise is generally a health benefit, vigorous exercise following exposure to an allergenic food may stimulate an allergic reaction for some people. Under stressful conditions, allergy symptoms seem to appear or worsen. In contrast, there is some scientific evidence that stress management and relaxation techniques may reduce symptoms in a variety of conditions that may be linked with food sensitivities, such as dermatitis. It has been demonstrated that serum levels of histamine can be altered by relaxation. Studies of asthmatics have shown that improved control of breathing through the practice of yoga or breathing exercises may contribute to the successful control of asthma. Research indicates that programs that include relaxation techniques can reduce pain in people with various forms of arthritis. Scientists have shown that relaxation, biofeedback, and stress management techniques are effective in reducing headache activity by 35–50 percent.

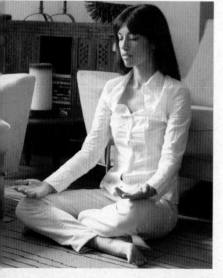

Stress management may reduce the symptoms of food sensitivities.

FOOD SENSITIVITY SYMPTOMS AND LOCATION

Location of Symptoms	Possible Symptoms
Digestive tract	belching, bloating, constipation, diarrhea, indigestion, nausea, stomach or abdominal pains, vomiting
Nervous system	depression, dizziness, fatigue, hyperactivity, irritability, lack of concentration, listlessness, migraines or other headaches, spots before the eyes
Respiratory tract	asthma (recurring attacks of labored breathing, chest constriction, coughing, and lung spasm); earache with fluid drainage; itchy, watery, reddened eyes; runny nose; sneezing; throat tightening (due to tissues swelling)
Skin and mucous membranes	eczema, hives, itching, redness, swelling of deeper tissues in the mouth and face
Other	dark circles under the eyes, muscle aches, sweating

Anaphylactic Reactions

Anaphylactic (originally meaning "no protection") reactions are severe, rapid reactions involving most organ systems of the body. In the most extreme cases, the reaction turns into anaphylactic shock, cardiac collapse, and death. Fortunately, protection is available for people who face the possibility of these serious, potential reactions. They must take great care to avoid their specific allergens and always carry with them a kit containing injectable adrenaline (epinephrine), typically in a delivery system called an EpiPen, and an oral antihistamine in case of accidental exposure. Foods most commonly implicated in anaphylactic reactions are peanuts, fish, shellfish, and tree nuts.

Causes of Food Allergies

Why Food Sensitivities Occur in One Person and Not Another

When we are diagnosed with food allergies, we often wonder, why me? Why do these adverse responses to food take place in some of us and not in others? The answer is linked to our genetics, history since birth (or even conception), and current lifestyles.

Inherited Patterns and Family Patterns We may inherit a tendency toward allergies in general. Furthermore, families pass along their eating patterns. For example, Mom may have learned from Grandma when to introduce certain foods during infancy, what the essentials are for stocking the family fridge and pantry, and which are the best recipes for chowder, omelets, or biscuits. It's not surprising that sensitivities to milk, eggs, or wheat would show up among family members. Also, we may inherit a greater vulnerability in one system of the body, such as the digestive system, skin, or nervous system. Family members share a home environment that has pollutants (such as cigarette smoke) or other factors that can increase our susceptibility to food sensitivities.

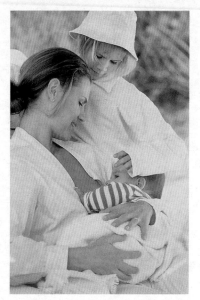

We also pass along habits of relaxation and reactions to stress that may moderate our symptoms. Even the types of bacteria in the intestine (which family members are likely to share) can influence our response to foods.

Breast-feeding a child, without any supplementary foods or formula, for the first six months of life is one course of action that is likely to reduce the risk of eczema, asthma, and gastrointestinal problems. This is a wise choice for infants whose parents, brothers, or sisters have allergies (and for all other infants, too). It's also important for a breast-feeding mother who has allergies herself to avoid the foods she is sensitive to. Breast milk provides protective factors, and it promotes the gradual maturation of the intestinal wall, increasing its ability to block allergens. For an allergy-prone infant who must receive formula, a hydrolyzed or partially hydrolyzed formula is likely to reduce the risk of an allergic reaction.

Breast milk provides protective factors that promote a strong digestive system.

Why Now? You may wonder why your reactions to particular foods have suddenly surfaced. For certain people, the food allergy, and even the symptoms, have been there all along, unnoticed. Sometimes a period of stress or overexposure to a certain food is enough to push

HOW MANY PEOPLE HAVE FOOD ALLERGIES?

To determine the number of people affected by food sensitivities, it is necessary to differentiate between true food allergies and food intolerance. According to some surveys, one person in three has reported that she or he has a food "allergy." Yet such self-reporting is not always confirmed when clinical trials or laboratory tests are conducted. The National Institutes of Health estimates that between 5 and 8 percent of children have true food allergies involving the immune system. The incidence of food allergies gradually decreases over time, reaching the adult rate of 1–2 percent in late childhood. If we include nonallergic food sensitivities (food intolerances), we could perhaps say that the number of people with some sort of food sensitivity is quite literally 100 percent. Who has not experienced some sort of adverse reaction to food, even a minor one, at one time or another? Yet with food intolerance, there are none of the objective laboratory indicators that occur with an immune response, where antibodies to a particular food protein can be seen in a blood sample. You may suspect that a reaction is linked with a certain food. However, when you have consumed a mixture of foods and beverages, it's hard to determine exactly what caused the reaction, and it may not happen every time or under all circumstances. Consequently, estimating the prevalence of food allergies is rather tricky.

Food intolerances seem to be more widespread than true food allergies. In one study that followed newborns to the age of three years, 28 percent of the infants were reported to have some sort of adverse reaction to a food. One-quarter of these were allergies that involved the immune system. Overall, one household in four adjusts its food habits due to food sensitivities.

symptoms from a slight undercurrent to a raging torrent. Odd as it seems, food allergies may come to our attention during a period in our lives when we have become more health conscious and have simply taken the time to observe our responses.

Food Allergies through Life

Most true food allergies are acquired during the first year of life. At one year of age, about 6–8 percent (or, by some reports, as many as 10 percent) of infants have developed food allergies. Since most gradually outgrow these reactions, about 1–2 percent of the adult population is affected by food allergy.

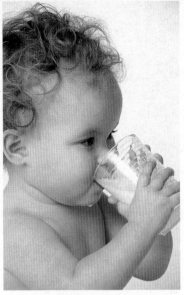

As many as 10 percent of infants may develop food allergies in their first year, but most outgrow them by adulthood.

If we experience allergies to certain foods (fish, peanuts, shellfish, or tree nuts) or a sensitivity to wheat gluten, the situation is typically with us for life, though variations occur. (For example, recent research has shown that one person in five may outgrow an allergy to peanuts.) Yet when it comes to other foods, some children or adults outgrow their reactions. One person in three loses his or her clinical reactivity after completely avoiding an allergen for one to two years. It seems that the immune system can forget to launch its adverse reaction to an allergen after there has been no contact for years. (However, those who are anaphylactic should not test this without medical supervision!)

Infants experience true allergies to various proteins in milk; these responses may be outgrown sometime during their next decade of life. A Danish study showed that 35 percent of infants with one food allergy went on to develop allergic reactions to other foods and that many developed allergies to inhaled substances. Males seem about twice as likely to develop food allergies as females. Considering all types of allergies, including those to inhaled substances and to food, if both parents are allergy free, there is a 5–15 percent chance of their child having allergies. If both parents have allergies, the risk jumps to 20 percent or as high as 60 percent.

Increased Frequency of Food Allergies Food allergies have increased at alarming rates in recent decades. For example, it is estimated that allergies have tripled during the last three decades in developed countries. Plausible theories for the cause of these changes span the spectrum from too much cleanliness in our lives, on the one hand, to the lack of it (in air quality, for example).

Hygiene theory. Scientists suggest that our overprotected and hygienic lifestyles may play a role in food allergies. According to this theory, children who are exposed to many foreign cells right from the start, as would be the case if they lived on a farm or in an environment closer to nature, develop an immune system that has turned its attention to effectively fighting off bacteria and viruses and away from fighting off food proteins. According to the theory, when children begin life in a clean, sanitized world, their immune systems may focus their reactions on food particles rather than on bacteria. It seems that having a few germs in our environment from the outset may stimulate our immune system to protect us properly.

Pollution. Though the hygiene theory presents an interesting perspective on lifestyles with few bacteria, some types of pollution seem to promote more food sensitivities. Early exposure to cigarette smoke, dust, pets, pollen, and other allergens can increase our risk of developing allergies in general.

Modern agricultural methods. Innovations such as genetic modification can produce protein molecules that are resistant to digestion. According to the Food and Agriculture Organization and the World Health Organization, these may be more likely to stimulate allergic reactions. Their international panel of experts has emphasized that all foods derived from biotechnology should be assessed for allergenic potential. However, this group lacks the power to enforce such a recommendation on food corporations, which conduct considerable food research. Yet the topic of long-term damage to human health due to genetically modified organisms (GMOs) or pesticides seems to attract relatively few of their research dollars.

Extensive use of pesticides and herbicides (which are, by definition, substances designed to destroy life) are being blamed for some of our reactions to foods. Some scientists and members of the public think that more research is needed about the novel foods, proteins, and chemicals that are constantly being added to our environment.

Skin testing for allergies. Though intradermal testing for food allergies is intended to penetrate only the top layer of skin, certain experts believe that skin testing for allergies may occasionally increase the range of foods to which a potentially allergic individual develops reactions. When a food allergen is allowed to reach the bloodstream through broken skin or, particularly, via injection, it bypasses mechanisms in the intestinal wall that nature has designed to protect us from the allergic response. Our natural protective mechanisms in the intestinal wall lead to oral tolerance for food proteins and the handling of foods without an allergic response.

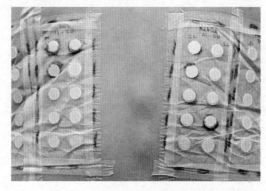

Skin-patch testing may actually increase the body's sensitivity to food allergens.

In a somewhat related mechanism, vaccines may trigger allergic responses. Influenza vaccines, used in flu shots, are grown on egg embryos and may contain a small amount of egg protein, which could potentially lead to an allergic response to egg. For more on this, see page 28.

Intestinal well-being. Our intestinal lining is beautifully designed to be a semipermeable membrane, like a sieve, that allows small molecules (such as the products of digestion) to pass through, while blocking larger molecules. These larger molecules may then travel through the intestine and be eliminated in feces. When functioning as intended, the intestinal lining (gut wall) is a barrier that prevents these large molecules from stimulating food allergenic reactions. Unfortunately, certain factors in our lifestyles can create and sustain unwanted "holes" in this barrier. Maintaining the health of the gut wall and avoiding a "leaky gut" (or restoring it to good health) may play a role in minimizing food allergies and preventing the development of further reactions to foods. A diet that includes fermented foods (or probiotic supplements) and the whole plant foods that sustain beneficial bacteria in the intestine can also be our ally.

Diagnosing Food Allergies . . . .

One of the most challenging and often frustrating aspects of having food allergies is the process of determining exactly which foods are causing our problems. Since we typically eat more than one food at a time, and often include a beverage, it can be very difficult to pinpoint which item or items in a meal or snack are the culprits. A reaction can occur immediately or as long as several hours after we eat an offending food. In addition, our bodies may not necessarily react the same way to a problem food every time we are exposed to it. This may be due to

13

variable qualities regarding the food itself, such as the food's freshness or origin. Further complicating matters, accompanying foods and beverages may influence the way our bodies react to certain foods. Reactions also may be due to our state of health or other factors. Illnesses, medications, stress, and even hormonal imbalances can change the degree to which a food triggers a reaction.

Laboratory Testing for Food Allergies

Historically, when people have suspected a food allergy, their doctors have referred them to an allergy specialist for testing. Whereas testing has some value as part of our overall detective work, alone its value is limited because of a high level of false positives (that is, we may test positive for a food allergy but experience no problems when we eat

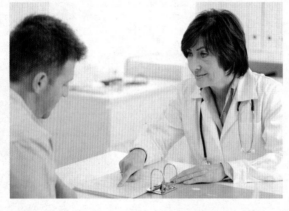

that food) and false negatives (that is, we may test negative for a food allergy even though we experience symptoms when we eat that food). Experts concur that for the most accurate results, a detailed medical history, family history, and physical exam should always accompany laboratory testing. When diagnosing a food allergy, the allergist should ask the following questions:

Traditional allergy specialists may suggest a variety of tests for a range of allergens.

- Which food or foods are suspected to have caused a reaction?
- What quantity of that food or foods has been shown to cause a reaction?
- What was the length of time between ingestion and the development of symptoms?
- How often has the food produced the symptoms?
- What other factors (such as exercise or alcohol) seem to affect the reaction?
- When was the last time a reaction occurred?

Traditional allergy testing does not reveal food sensitivities or intolerances, only IgE-mediated allergies (that is, sensitivities that cause the immune system to react). In tracking down the culprit foods, it is important to remember that we and our doctors or other health professionals must work as a team. Our awareness about the reactions we experience and the conditions surrounding them is a tremendously important part of the detective work.

Skin Tests

Skin tests are usually the first approach used by allergists. There are three types of skin tests:

- Prick test. The prick test is the most common skin test. It involves placing a drop of liquid containing the test allergen on the skin. This is followed by a skin prick underneath the drop.
- Scratch test. During the scratch test the skin is lightly scraped and the liquid is dropped on the site.
- Intradermal test. For the intradermal test, the liquid containing the allergen is injected just under the top layer of the skin with a syringe.

The allergist looks for redness and swelling at the site, as this is considered the basis for a positive result in each case, although this result is suggestive rather than conclusive. To clarify the diagnosis, a positive test can be followed by a food challenge, if desired (see page 16).

Most experts agree that skin testing is only one piece of the puzzle because it has many limitations, including the following:

- Skin testing produces false positive and false negative results.
- The skin and the intestine are two separate organs, and the cells of each may react differently to the same protein.
- The food extracts used for the test may lack the proteins that cause a reaction when the food is eaten.
- Patients with skin conditions, such as eczema, are not good candidates for skin tests.
- Skin tests, particularly the intradermal test, may cause a systemic and/or anaphylactic reaction.
- There is concern among some experts that intradermal testing could potentially be the initial trigger for a food allergy.

It is important to know that skin tests are not useful for detecting allergies to foods that cause a delayed reaction. This is a significant limitation. Skin testing for a large number of foods is rarely necessary or helpful. If you decide to go for testing, be wary of clinics that suggest skin testing for twenty to thirty foods. Testing should be tailored to you, based on your symptoms, history, and state of health.

Blood tests. Blood tests are simpler and safer than skin tests, but their value is similarly limited by false results. The most common blood tests are the RAST (an abbreviation for radioallergosorbent test) and ELISA (short for enzyme-linked immunosorbent assay). These are less invasive than skin tests because, although a blood sample is drawn, the test itself takes place outside the body and therefore does not pose the risk of a reaction. These tests measure the presence of food-specific IgE (the globulin protein that our immune system generates for that specific food protein) in the blood. The results are typically provided in a scale of numerical values; the higher the number, the higher the circulating levels of IgG (scales vary per lab). However, this does not guarantee the presence of a true food allergy, and a negative test result does not necessarily rule out the diagnosis of an allergy.

For both skin and blood tests, it is common for a patient to test positive to several members of the same botanical family of plant foods or animal species, yet they may have a true sensitivity to only one food in the family, so all are not necessarily allergens. This is one reason why positive tests should be viewed with a degree of skepticism; the un-necessary elimination of foods can result in nutrient deficiencies, increased social challenges, and decreased quality of life.

Finally, novel approaches to testing are constantly being developed, so ask your health provider which test may be the most appropriate for your situation.

Dietary Approaches for the Diagnosis of Food Allergy
Practitioner-Guided Food Challenges

The oral food challenge is the most reliable test known for food allergies. Simply stated, this test involves the elimination of specific foods (suspected food culprits) from the diet for a certain period of time (during which symptoms may subside), followed by a "test dose" of this food to see if symptoms develop. Some practitioners take this procedure one step further by prescribing the double-blind, placebo-controlled food challenge (DBPCFC), considered the gold standard. In the DBPCFC, the food being tested is administered in such as way that neither the practitioner nor the patient knows whether the possible food culprit or a placebo has been given. If symptoms occur only with the food, the test result is positive.

Keeping a record of everything you eat and when symptoms occur can help pinpoint foods that cause sensitivities.

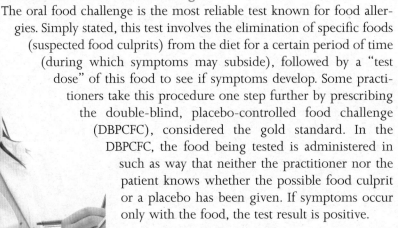

Oral Food Challenges An oral food challenge may be conducted by a health practitioner (as summarized above) or by oneself. Done properly, an oral food challenge takes quite a bit of time and effort, but the rewards of good health certainly are worth the energy expended in the quest to identify problem foods. The oral food challenge involves three steps: (1) the use of a food diary, (2) an elimination diet, and (3) a challenge with a suspected food culprit.

Food diary. Detailed food diaries often prove successful in providing the clues necessary to pinpoint problem foods. A food diary should involve a detailed list of all the foods eaten, the quantity of each food, the ingredient lists of prepared foods when possible, and a notation of the time the food was consumed. Foods placed in the mouth but not swallowed, such as chewing gum, must be included as well. Also important is a record of any symptoms and the times they occur. A food diary should be kept for as long as possible before, during, and after the elimination-diet phase. It may be helpful to list any activities or recent circumstances that could be involved, for example, your current state of health, including any illnesses; your exercise regimen; any medications and/or supplements you are taking; and any particularly stressful events in your life.

Elimination diet. During the elimination diet you should eat as you normally do, except that you should completely avoid the food or foods that you suspect are causing problems. It is imperative that you eliminate all possible sources of these foods. For example, if you suspect a soy allergy, you must avoid all foods containing soy, including those that may have "hidden" sources of soy, such as flavor enhancers. Typically, four to six weeks of complete avoidance of the suspected foods is recommended. For details on how to perform your own elimination diet, see pages 18–22.

17

FOOD DIARY CHECKLIST

In your diary, be sure to include the following:

√ Everything you eat, drink, and place in your mouth, listing each item by the date and time of day it is consumed

√ All the ingredients in the recipes you prepare

√ All the ingredients on the labels of any packaged foods you eat

√ All the ingredients in foods eaten away from home (limit these foods during your test, if possible)

√ Any medications, prescribed or over-the-counter

√ Any supplements (herbs, vitamins, minerals)

√ Your state of health and any illnesses you are experiencing

√ Any symptoms, including the time and length of the reaction

A challenge with a suspected food culprit. This challenge involves consuming the suspect food, whether in a capsule, extracted and placed in a beverage, hidden in other foods, or simply eaten in the regular manner. If this is done in a clinic, a clinician will observe whether symptoms develop. If you are investigating your response to more than one food, it is important that, after four to six weeks of avoidance of all suspected food culprits, you gradually reintroduce the eliminated foods one at a time. Several days should elapse between each food challenge to allow sufficient time for symptoms to develop and subside, and for the test foods to exit the system.

Do-It-Yourself Elimination Diet and Food Challenge

Whether or not you decide to visit a clinic to undergo formal laboratory testing, if you suspect that food is at the root of your poor health, one powerful strategy you can undertake yourself is the elimination diet and food challenge. This can be done on your own or with the assistance of a registered dietitian, who can help you meet your nutrient requirements while you are eliminating a number of potentially problematic foods. She or he also may help you identify hidden sources of the foods you are avoiding. If you have had a severe reaction to a food in the past, never try a food challenge involving this food without professional supervision.

Step 1: Your food diary. You may need to modify the traditional elimination diet used by allergists, because nonallergic food intolerances tend to have more subtle effects on the body than true allergies, and these effects tend to be related to the quantity of the food that is consumed. Therefore, we recommend that you keep a very detailed food diary that includes all foods and ingredients that you consume, and a list of the symptoms, feelings, and physical reactions that you experience, bearing in mind that symptoms may arise immediately after, several

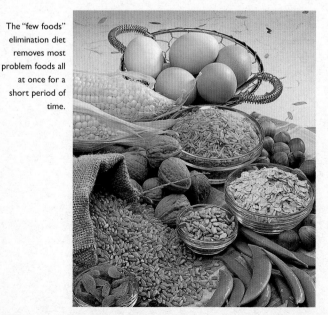

The "few foods" elimination diet removes most problem foods all at once for a short period of time.

18

"FEW FOODS" ELIMINATION DIET

General Protocol

√ Wash and cook foods with distilled water only.

√ Use glass, iron, or aluminum cookware and utensils; avoid stainless steel, plastic, and nonstick-coated materials.

√ Consult your doctor about medications that must be continued versus those that can be avoided during the diet.

Permitted Foods

Beverages: distilled water, juice from allowed fruits and vegetables

Condiments: non-iodized sea salt

Desserts: pudding made from tapioca or rice and sweetened with the juice of allowed fruits (no milk or eggs)

Fruits: cranberries, pears (and the juice from cranberries and pears)

Grains: millet, rice, tapioca

Legumes: dried lentils (rinsed well and boiled)

Oils: canola, sunflower (select the cold-pressed variety)

Vegetables: lettuce, parsnips, squash, sweet potatoes, yams

Note: Agar, a bland sea vegetable, often called "vegetable gelatin" because of its jelling abilities, may be used as a thickener for puddings. Agar is available in natural food stores and Asian markets. It must be simmered in a liquid, preferably water, on the stovetop for 5–10 minutes, or in the microwave, until it is dissolved. It will thicken more as it cools. To jell about 2 cups of liquid, use 2 tablespoons of agar flakes or 1 1/2 to 2 teaspoons of agar powder.

Source: Adapted from *Dealing With Food Allergies* by J. V. Joneja.

hours after, and several days after you eat a trigger food. Keep this diary for at least two weeks before you make any changes to your diet, and continue to keep it throughout the next two phases of the challenge.

Step 2: Elimination phase. Next, you must choose which food or foods to eliminate from your diet during the elimination phase. The foods you select will depend on your symptoms, your diet, and your past experiences. Your diary and past history may provide clues to help you pinpoint the foods that are causing your discomfort. Keep in mind that you may need to eliminate the suspicious food or foods for several weeks before you notice a change in your symptoms. It is possible that you will initially feel worse after eliminating a problem food; this may mean that your body is readjusting to a new state while it is no longer dealing with that food. If this is the case, after a couple of days the symptoms should subside. Be sure to continue to keep your detailed diary during the elimination phase.

For your elimination diet you can take one of the following two approaches:

1. Eliminate foods or groups of foods based on your suspicions that they are the root of your problem. This diet is typically followed for about four weeks.

2. Practice the "few foods" approach. This involves the elimination of practically every food that may cause a reaction, leaving your diet stripped down to just a few hypoallergenic foods. This diet is followed for only a short period of time because such restricted food intake cannot provide complete nutrition and may actually suppress the immune system. Due to the difficulty of sustaining the "few foods" diet for more than a few days, and because of the risk of nutrient deficiency, we recommend the first approach in most cases. The "few foods" approach is best suited for those with particularly severe symptoms who are unable to identify problem foods using traditional allergy testing or a regular elimination diet. If you would like to take this approach, be sure to discuss it with your health-care provider. The "few foods" diet is not nutritionally adequate for extended periods of time and should be followed for no more than ten days (usually seven days is sufficient).

If you follow the "few foods" elimination diet for a short period, you will discover that, although this diet is limited, even one type of grain, plus a few fruits and vegetables, still allow for variety in textures and flavors. Crunchy rice cakes (plain or salted) can be spread with pear sauce; cream of rice cereal and puffed rice are tasty with cranberries and juice; rice flakes make a topping for a cranberry-pear crumble; and rice salad can be dotted with chopped vegetables. Rice noodles or rice vermicelli can be served with cooked vegetables or used in a vegetable soup. Rice-paper wrappers, available from Asian food markets, can be dipped in cold water (to soften them) and then wrapped around a mixture of cooked rice and chopped vegetables to form a sandwich. Winter squash (hard-shell squash) with the seeds removed can be stuffed with cooked grains and baked. Cooked brown rice can be combined with four times

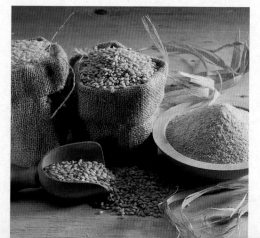

Brown rice can be used in crackers, hot cereal, salads, pasta, and even milk to provide variety in a diet.

20

as much water and blended to make a milk. (After blending, let the mixture rest for one hour, and then strain and refrigerate.) Several types of rice are available: brown rice (short grain, medium grain, and long grain), basmati, Arborio, jasmine, and glutinous (sweet) rice. You can also find exotic and fragrant red, brown, and black rice. Brown rice contains B vitamins, iron, zinc, and other trace minerals, as well as fiber. About 9 percent of the calories in rice come from protein. White rice is less nutritious.

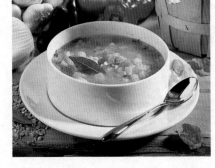

Lentils are an excellent source of protein and complex carbohydrates.

Lentils can be made into a variety of soups, cooked and served alone as a main dish, or cooked along with the allowed vegetables and grains. Mashed lentils mixed with mashed cooked vegetables, a little fruit juice, and salt make a tasty spread for rice crackers. Lentils are an excellent source of protein, and the complex carbohydrates they contain will help you maintain consistent blood sugar levels, providing energy between meals.

If you plan on trying the "few foods" approach, we recommend that you take a multivitamin-mineral supplement during the elimination and reintroduction phases. (Check the supplement's label for allergenic ingredients.)

Most people will be successful in pinpointing problem foods using the first approach (that is, by eliminating a specific food or foods that seem to be problematic). Depending on your symptoms, it might be wise not to eliminate too many foods all at once. Avoiding too many healthful foods may rob you of essential nutrients, leaving you feeling sluggish and fatigued and making it increasingly difficult to pinpoint the original source of your symptoms. However, if you have multiple food sensitivities, the symptoms may not go away if you eliminate only one food at a time. (This is typical of migraine headache sufferers; symptoms are often triggered by several foods, not just one food.) Because of these competing issues, there is no single approach that is suitable for everyone. One solution may be to try eliminating one food at a time in an attempt to pinpoint the culprit; but if this does not work, eliminate several foods you may suspect are causing your symptoms. If neither of these approaches is successful, the "few foods" elimination diet is the next step. Based on your personal experiences, reactions, and food diary, you may already suspect which food or foods are the offenders.

Step 3: Your food challenge. The most important thing to remember when attempting your food challenge is that you must reintroduce only one eliminated food at a time. Except for the one food being challenged, your diet should be exactly the same as it was

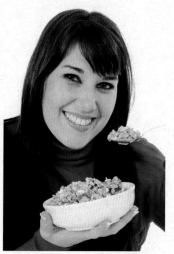

during the elimination phase. If you reintroduce several eliminated foods at once, it will be nearly impossible to determine which of the foods is the culprit.

Here's the recommended approach for initiating the challenge. At breakfast, reintroduce a small amount of only one of the foods you eliminated and wait until lunchtime to see if your symptoms return. If you don't have any reaction, try a larger portion of the same food at lunch. Again, wait it out until dinnertime and try once more with a still larger portion. If you still have no adverse symptoms, wait two days and repeat the process with your next test food. For each food tested, the day after the first test do not consume any more of the test food until the entire testing is completed. Keep in mind that you may experience a delayed reaction. If you do experience a reaction at any point during the test, discontinue the food. Continue to record in your food diary all the foods you have eaten and any symptoms experienced.

If you are eliminating a group of foods, such as tree nuts, this test may reveal that you can tolerate only some foods but not others in the group (for example, almonds may cause symptoms but pecans do not). You may also discover that you have a tolerance for a certain amount of a food before you begin to experience symptoms—for example, one-half ounce of cashews can be tolerated, but symptoms begin to appear if you eat an ounce or more. Using this careful approach should lead to success in identifying problem foods.

You may find that you feel so much better on your elimination diet that you don't wish to reintroduce problem foods; after all, why make yourself sick again after achieving remission? This is perfectly okay if you have eliminated only one food. If you have eliminated many foods, it is important to figure out which one or ones are triggering your symptoms. It is also important to maintain variety in your diet while removing the foods that are causing your problems.

Hidden Culprits . . . .

When we have food sensitivities, or when we care or cook for those who do, we soon discover that problematic ingredients can sneak into our diets in all sorts of unexpected and mysterious ways. Taking precautions to avoid these hidden culprits is important, and for some of us this detective work can be life saving.

Cross-contamination can occur in commercial food prep kitchens.

Cross-Contamination

A common scenario occurs when people accidentally consume a "hidden" substance that has contaminated an otherwise safe food. This is known as cross-contamination. This can happen, for example, if the same serving utensil is used for different foods. At a salad bar, restaurant buffet, or potluck meal we may have little idea where the scoop was sitting a few minutes before we picked it up. Cross-contamination occurs at deli counters and sandwich shops when the same knife or slicer is used for meat, cheese, seafood, hard-boiled eggs, and vegetables. It also occurs when a restaurant or fast-food shop uses the same oil to fry various items.

Cross-contamination can take place when a manufacturing plant uses the same equipment to make or package various products (such as ice cream and milk-free sorbet, milk chocolate and dairy-free dark chocolate, or soymilk and cow's milk) without adequately cleaning the equipment between runs. It can happen when gluten-free grains and gluten-containing grains are processed in the same mill or cereal plant. Fortunately, some companies take a great deal of care to avoid this sort of cross-contamination; however, many do not. People with serious food allergies are wise to become familiar with companies whose practices they can trust.

Ingredient Substitution

Another source of concern with manufactured food products is substituting ingredients. This can occur when there is a shortage of an ingredient and a manufacturer makes a temporary replacement (such as using peanut oil instead of 100 percent corn oil) or when a company permanently changes ingredients without making this clear on the label.

23

Consumer Error

Mistakes take place when consumers assume that a brand of food has similar formulations for a range of products (such as a line of soups, cereals, veggie burgers, or nondairy milks). To avoid unwanted milk or dairy proteins, soy, nuts, wheat gluten, or other allergens, it is crucial to read all product labels. Companies change their formulations from time to time, so it's wise to check even those products you purchase regularly.

Food Packaging

It is possible that a nonallergenic food is packed in material that contains a food allergen. For example, some manufacturers use starch dust to prevent packaging from sticking to itself. Others may use foil coated with a wheat ingredient. While it is rare that packaging material causes an allergic reaction, highly sensitive individuals should be aware of this possibility.

Misleading Labels

The Food Allergy Labeling and Consumer Protection Act (enacted in 2006) mandates that the labels of foods containing major food allergens (milk, eggs, fish, crustacean shellfish, peanuts, tree nuts, wheat, and soy)—even tiny amounts—declare the allergen in plain language. However, mistakes happen, and some companies have not successfully complied, so exercise caution with packaged foods, particularly brands that are not well known.

Because food-manufacturing practices vary throughout the world, imported foods can be a concern. Also, unknown ingredients may be present in raw materials. Fortunately, international food producers are becoming increasingly aware of the potential seriousness of errors.

Specific Allergens and How to Stay Safe . . . .

Milk and Dairy Products

Our friends and acquaintances may tell us of milk "allergies" in their families. Yet their symptoms and the milk components that trigger their reactions may differ considerably. Some individuals, particularly infants and children, experience true allergic reactions to any of the more than twenty-five proteins in milk, whereas adults tend to be intolerant to the sugar (lactose) in milk.

Allergic reactions to milk most frequently affect the skin and the digestive system, although reactions can also occur in other parts of the body. Cheese and ice cream can trigger migraine headaches. Milk may trigger or worsen asthma attacks. For some children, milk consumption is linked with restlessness and difficulty sleeping. Milk-related inflammation along the intestine may induce fecal blood loss, resulting in iron deficiency. Furthermore, damage to cells along the intestinal wall can lead to the insufficient absorption of nutrients.

Lactose intolerance, which is *not* an allergic reaction, occurs when the amount of dairy products (specifically, the milk sugar lactose that is in the dairy products) consumed exceeds the ability of the intestinal enzyme lactase to digest, or break down, the lactose. Undigested lactose remains in the intestinal tract and causes water to be drawn into the intestine, resulting in abdominal distension and bloating. When lactose reaches the lower intestine, the bacteria that inhabit this area feast on the undigested sugar, producing gas and acid. This produces cramps, flatulence, and often diarrhea. Lactose intolerance does not affect the skin or respiratory system, as a true milk allergy can.

We can expect that 80 percent or more of people with cow's milk allergy will show a similar response to goat's milk because most of the proteins in the two milks are similar. Lactose is present in the milk of all species. Therefore, goat's milk cannot be substituted for cow's milk in cases of lactose intolerance and is seldom suitable for those with allergies to milk protein.

Although it's easy to avoid obvious dairy products such as milk and cheese, buying prepared foods without dairy products as an ingredient can be more of a challenge. We know to look for the word "milk" on ingredient lists, but dairy by-products can also come in various disguises. Extracted milk proteins that are added to foods may be listed as "casein," "caseinate," "whey," "lactalbumin," or "lactoglobulin"; hydrolysates of these may also be allergenic. Though some proteins in milk are altered by heating, others are not and may trigger reactions. Caramel coloring and caramel flavorings are sometimes made from burnt lactose, and "natural flavorings"

Buying prepared foods without dairy products can be a challenge.

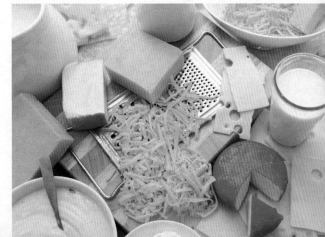

and brown sugar flavoring can be milk based. Despite the similarity in name, lactic acid, lactate, and lactylate do not contain milk and do not need to be eliminated from the diet. Nevertheless, a label listing of "lactic acid starter culture" may indicate that the product contains some milk.

Milk and its derivatives are found in a large variety of processed foods. Some are fairly obvious, such as cream, skim milk, milk chocolate, cheese, ice cream, yogurt, and many baked goods. Less obvious and occasionally surprising are "nondairy" creamers and some brands of dark chocolate. Margarine often contains milk protein, such as whey. Many soy cheeses contain casein, as this milk protein allows the product to melt well and have a characteristic cheese "stretch." Check the ingredient list on some soy products, such as soy cheeses, even if they are marked as dairy free or milk free. Lactose, which may contain residual milk protein, often is used as a filler in the manufacture of medicinal capsules and pill tablets. Ingredient lists are usually available from deli counters and restaurants for foods that don't come with ingredient labeling.

In hard cheeses and yogurt the amount of lactose is reduced compared with the amount in the original cow's milk. Very little lactose is present in butter and in margarine that contains whey. Products such as Lactaid and Lacteeze milks still contain milk protein and may contain a small amount of lactose. Some people consume lactase tablets along with milk to help them break down milk sugar. However, people who are allergic to molds and fungus should use caution with these pills, as they may react to the fungus used to manufacture the lactase enzyme or to one of the additives in the tablets.

Living Without Dairy: *Restaurants and traveling.* Allergies to milk protein need not prevent you from enjoying a wonderful meal when you're out on the town or traveling.

Chinese and Japanese restaurants offer many delicious dishes made without dairy products.

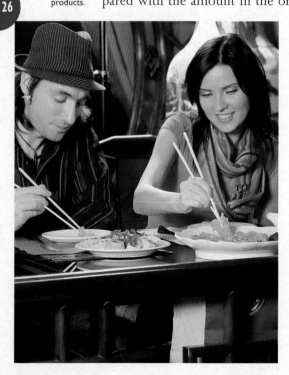

26

Chinese, Thai, and Japanese restaurants can accommodate you very well. Middle Eastern and African restaurants are likely to have many dairy-free entrées. Though usually not mentioned on the menu, ghee (clarified butter) is often used in Indian restaurants as a base for recipes, even for seemingly dairy-free vegetable dishes, so check with your server. Vegan restaurants serve no animal products and are among the safest places for people with milk allergies. Many vegetarian restaurants offer a number of nondairy items. (For restaurant choices, check www.happycow.net.)

Most restaurants take care to deal with special requests for people with food allergies, so let your server know about your needs. Often dairy is used in preparing a dish, though it may not be mentioned on the menu. It is important that your server check with the chef to determine which items are safe for you. In some cases, the butter, cheese, or dairy-based sauce can simply be omitted from a recipe. Breakfast can be the most challenging meal. When traveling or visiting others, it helps to take along powdered or fluid nondairy milk to add to cereal or to a hot beverage, such as tea or coffee. Juice, such as apple juice, tastes good on cereal, too. When traveling with an allergic child, be sure to take a few favorite beverages and foods.

Food preparation without dairy. In recent years, natural food stores and mainstream supermarkets have expanded their offerings of nondairy milks, cheeses, sour creams, puddings, and frozen desserts. Dairy-free margarines, such as several varieties of Earth Balance, Soy Garden, and Spectrum Spread, are available. As long as you avoid the reduced-calorie varieties, you can expect these products to taste delicious; they melt beautifully and can be used for cooking and baking,

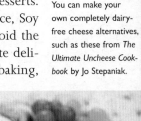

You can make your own completely dairy-free cheese alternatives, such as these from *The Ultimate Uncheese Cookbook* by Jo Stepaniak.

substituted measure for measure for stick margarine or butter. The quality and flavor of many of these products makes it a pleasure to go dairy free.

Fortunately, vegan cheese alternatives (those that contain no milk products, including casein) are readily available. The taste and texture of commercial vegan cheese products have been steadily improving. We find that the best-tasting "uncheeses" are homemade. For recipes, try *The Ultimate Uncheese Cookbook* by Jo Stepaniak.

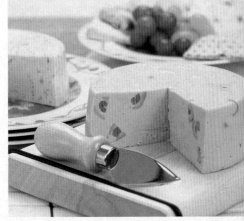

Being Well Nourished Without Dairy

Cow's milk and milk products constitute an entire food group on some national food guides, but this is largely due to the powerful dairy lobbies in these countries. These items are not essential to human nutrition. In many parts of the world, dairy products are not on the food guides and are not part of everyday meals. All of the nutrients in dairy products are readily available in a variety of other foods.

Infants. Because liquids are the mainstay of life for infants, the primary beverages for those with milk allergies must be considered carefully, and your health-care provider should be consulted on this. Breast milk is always best. For bottle-fed infants, a hydrolyzed or partially hydrolyzed formula may be necessary. Hypoallergenic milk-based formulas have been used as milk replacements for infants with dairy allergies. However, hypoallergenic milk formulas are not necessarily nonallergenic, and sensitive children may have a reaction to them, depending on the particular formula.

Children. For children aged two and older who can tolerate soy, fortified soymilks can be used; the amounts of calcium, vitamin D, and protein are similar to those in cow's milk. Compared with whole cow's milk, soymilk is higher in iron and a little lower in fat. Some soymilks contain added vitamin B_{12} and riboflavin; in Canada, zinc is added as well. Other nondairy milks, such as rice, almond, hemp, and oat, are often fortified and provide a pleasant variety of flavors. Note that 1 cup (250 milliliters) of soymilk contains 7–9 grams of protein, whereas rice milk (fortified or not) provides only about 0.5 grams of protein per cup. If your best option for a child or teen is fortified rice milk, it is important that the diet contains plenty of other protein sources.

Eggs

Eggs contain a number of proteins to which we may be allergic; most are found in the white part of the egg. Some of these proteins are heat stable and are allergenic whether they are raw or cooked. Egg consumption by an allergic person can result in severe or anaphylactic reactions, especially in children under seven, and should be carefully avoided by those with this risk. Someone with a proven egg allergy should avoid both the white and yolk, unless it is established that one or the other can be tolerated safely. Furthermore, even when the white and yolk are separated, there is likely to be some cross-contamination. Eggs from various species contain similar proteins, so those who are allergic to chicken eggs should also avoid eggs from ducks, turkeys,

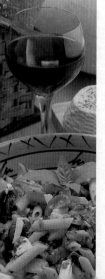

Eggs are a common ingredient in many prepared foods, such as baked goods, many pastas and noodles, and even wines.

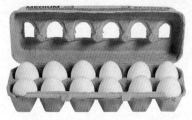

and other birds, unless their safety has been established. Because the blood of the hen is sometimes found in her eggs, some people who are allergic to chicken flesh may need to avoid chicken eggs as well.

A variety of terms in a food label may indicate the presence of egg protein. Check for egg as part of a phrase, such as "dried egg." The term "ovo" comes from the Latin word for egg and is a clue to its presence, as it is often used as part of a word. In some cases, even though food-labeling laws prohibit it, the ingredient itself is not mentioned on a label; instead, we are told the function that the egg performs in the product, such as "binder," "emulsifier," or "coagulant."

The proteins in eggs that cause the most allergic reactions are found in the white part of the egg.

Many wines are clarified with egg whites, though the label will not indicate this. In most manufactured food products that contain lecithin, the lecithin used is derived from soy, but occasionally the source may be egg. Provitamin A, which is extracted from eggs, may be used and described simply as a colorant, but it is not yet known whether this can cause an allergic reaction. In addition to food products, egg proteins also are found in some cosmetics, shampoos, nutritional supplements, and pharmaceuticals, such as laxatives. Influenza vaccines, used in flu shots, are grown on egg embryos and may contain a small amount of egg protein.

Living Without Eggs: *Restaurants and traveling.* Avoiding obvious egg dishes, such as omelets, quiche, or eggnog, is a simple matter. However, a small amount of egg is an ingredient in many manufactured foods, so allergic individuals must inquire. Eggs are a staple in most baked goods, so you'll find them in cakes, doughnuts, fancy pastries, glazed rolls, glazed nuts, and some biscuits, breads, and cookies. Eggs are often an ingredient in pastas (especially homemade and fresh pastas), commercial sauce mixes, soups, sausages, meat loaves and meat jellies, marshmallows, marzipan, icings, fancy ice creams, and other foods. Wines, soft drinks, and consommés often are clarified with egg whites. Avoid batter-coated items, such as vegetable tempura in Japanese restaurants. In Chinese restaurants, noodles typically contain eggs. Avoid buying fried foods from restaurants and vendors that use the same frying surface for preparing multiple types of food. Vegetarian and vegan restaurants often have delicious breakfast options and eggless entrées, baked goods, and desserts. To find restaurants in your neighborhood or when traveling, visit www.happycow.net.

Food preparation without eggs. Read package labels carefully. In recipes, eggs provide a source of liquid; egg protein acts as a binder to hold together cakes, cookies, and burgers; and beaten eggs provide lightness by helping to incorporate air in little bubbles. It's a simple matter to replace eggs with a similar amount of liquid or wet foods, such as juice, nondairy milk, water, applesauce, or mashed bananas. In many hypoallergenic recipes for baked goods, nonallergenic binders, such as xanthan gum or guar gum, are used. Ground flaxseeds mixed with water also make an excellent replacement for eggs in baked items, pancakes, and waffles. As a bonus, the flaxseeds will boost your intake of omega-3 fatty acids. Use 1 tablespoon (15 milliliters) of ground flaxseeds to 3 tablespoons (45 milliliters) of water for each egg. For leavening, baking powder or baking soda are very effective. (Baking soda requires the presence of something sour, like vinegar or lemon juice, for its leavening action to work.) It's helpful to know that when we just omit the one or two eggs called for in some of our favorite baked goods, such as muffins, the end result typically turns out just as well, even without any replacements.

Being Well Nourished Without Eggs Eggs provide protein, several vitamins (such as folate, pantothenic acid, riboflavin, and vitamin B_{12}), and iron. However, these nutrients can easily be supplied by other foods, so avoiding eggs should not create any risk of deficiency.

Soy

Soybeans are legumes and are botanically related to other legumes, including peanuts and beans. Nevertheless, people who cannot tolerate soy frequently can eat other legumes without adverse reactions. In skin tests for allergies, a legume mix (such as peanuts, soy, and green peas) is often used. If a reaction occurs, the test results are often mistakenly interpreted to mean that the patient is sensitive to all legumes. In truth, the proteins in various legumes differ, and claiming a sensitivity to all legumes based on a reaction to an individual legume can lead to an unnecessarily restrictive diet. Some clinics and labs test for individual beans, peas, and lentils, and it is worthwhile to

People who cannot tolerate soy can eat other legumes without adverse reactions.

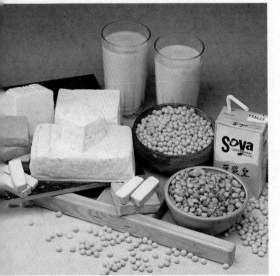

ask about this so that more of these highly nutritious foods can be included in your diet.

Soy allergy is most frequently seen in infants. It is less common than allergies to eggs, milk, peanuts, tree nuts, fish, and wheat, and is frequently outgrown by the age of three. Fortunately, soy rarely causes anaphylaxis. But unfortunately, people with soy allergy or intolerance may suffer from varying degrees of asthma, stuffy nose, intestinal inflammation and discomfort, and skin reactions. Because symptoms may be mild (but aggravating nonetheless), it is possible to go for years without realizing that soy is the root of poor health.

Soy and soy derivatives are found in a great number of processed foods.

In the processed-food industry there has been almost unlimited use of soy and soy derivatives, making it a particularly ubiquitous and menacing hidden allergen. As with many other food allergens, reactions may occur with exposure to very small quantities of soy protein. Some sources of soy are fairly obvious and easy to avoid: soy-based veggie burgers, soymilk, tofu, tempeh, soy flour, soy oil, and the beans themselves. However, because of the wide variety of ways that soy is used in the manufacture of various foods—including as a texturizer, emulsifier, and protein filler—eliminating it completely can be a challenge. Even though food manufacturers are now required by law to declare the word "soy" on any soy-derived product (such as "hydrolyzed protein" or "lecithin"), not all labels are compliant.

Soy protein isolate and concentrate are commonly used to emulsify fat in food products. Therefore, they may be present in ice cream, mayonnaise, and a variety of other liquid fat- or oil-containing foods. They also may be used in soymilk and as a protein concentrate added to "health foods" and high-protein bars, powders, and beverages. Other foods that may contain soy include puréed baby foods, cereals, margarine, and white and brown bread (for example, whole wheat, rye, or pumpernickel). Additional uses of soy in the processed-food industry include soy-based and other nondairy ice creams, nondairy cheeses, textured vegetable protein, meat extenders, and vegetarian meat alternatives.

Soybean flour often is added to cereal-grain flours and is used extensively in the baking industry. The majority of commercial breads contain some amount of soy flour. Baby foods, biscuits, cakes, and pastries may also contain soy flour. Fermented soybeans are commonly used in the preparation of soy sauce and worcestershire sauce, and fermented soy products in various forms are widely used in Asian cuisines.

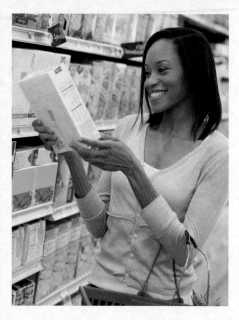

Soybean oil has many uses and can be found in baby foods, margarines, salad dressings, and many nonfood items (such as glue, linoleum, paint, plastics, and soap). Labels should be but are not always clear about the presence of soy; often "vegetable oil" is an oil blend containing soy. Although it was initially thought that soybean oil was safe for soy-sensitive individuals, soy proteins may be present in the oil, depending on the extraction process and the oil's purity. Cold-pressed or expeller-processed soy oil is more likely to contain soy protein than soy oil that has undergone the hot-solvent extraction process. The vitamin E in many multivitamin supplements is derived from soy.

Read food labels carefully—you're likely to find hidden sources of soy in processed foods.

32

Living Without Soy: *Restaurants and traveling.* Check out websites of chain restaurants; many post allergy information and will indicate which restaurant items are free of soy. However, beware of busy restaurants, which are a common source of cross-contamination. If you are very sensitive to soy, it is best to avoid chain or fast-food restaurants. Your best bets are restaurants that make everything from scratch. Raw-food restaurants can certainly accommodate you. Indian, Italian, and Middle Eastern eateries may be able to accommodate you, but Chinese, Japanese, Korean, and Thai restaurants rely heavily on soy ingredients and are therefore best avoided. Diners and American eateries often use soy oil for frying; ask the manager if you can get foods that do not depend on soy oil or other soy derivatives.

Food preparation without soy. Soy is a relatively recent addition to the cuisine of Western countries. Consequently, it is less commonly used as a basic ingredient in recipes and home-prepared foods compared with eggs and dairy products. When you shop, read ingredient labels carefully. You're more likely to encounter hidden sources of soy in foods prepared outside the home and in processed foods.

Being Well Nourished Without Soy Soy is a major source of protein in many vegetarian diets and a considerable source of fat (via soybean oil) in most diets. Some excellent soy-free, high-protein ingredients for main dishes include beans, lentils, peas, and wheat gluten. Grains, nuts, and seeds provide protein as well.

Fortunately, giving up soy oil may be a blessing because much of the soy oil found in processed foods is hydrogenated, a form best avoided by everyone. The most healthful sources of fats are whole foods such as nuts, seeds, avocados and olives.

If you are unable to tolerate both dairy and soy products, good toppings for cereal are almond milk, other nut milks, and rice milk. Look for varieties with added calcium, vitamin D, and vitamin B_{12}.

Formula-fed infants who cannot tolerate formulas made with cow's milk or soy may be given Similac Alimentum or Enfamil Nutramigen formulas, which are hypoallergenic.

Peanuts

Peanuts are one of the most allergenic foods and the leading cause of severe allergic reactions in the United States and Canada. The prevalence of peanut allergy has climbed dramatically over the past few years: an estimated 1.5 million Americans are peanut sensitive. Peanut allergy is outgrown about 20 percent of the time and occurs more commonly among people with asthma, skin conditions, or other food allergies. About one-third of peanut-sensitive individuals have severe, life-threatening reactions to peanuts. People with peanut allergies often are concerned about possible reactions from tree nuts; however, tree nuts are botanically unrelated to the peanut, which is a legume. It is estimated that 25–35 percent of people with peanut allergy also have a sensitivity to tree nuts. If tree nuts are tolerated and desired, sources that are not contaminated with peanuts should be sought, as nuts can make important contributions to a healthful diet, including protein, calories, vitamin E, trace minerals, and protective phytochemicals.

People with peanut allergies do not always have a sensitivity to tree nuts.

The most notable symptom of peanut allergy is anaphylaxis. However, people with a less severe sensitivity to peanuts may experience asthma, hives, nausea, stuffy nose, watery eyes, or wheezing. Families with food allergies should wait until a child is at least three years old before introducing peanut products; the decision should be dependent upon the family history of food allergies and whether the child suffers from asthma, intestinal disorders, or skin problems. An infant may react to peanut proteins in the mother's breast milk; if that happens, the mother should avoid peanut-containing foods until after the child has been weaned.

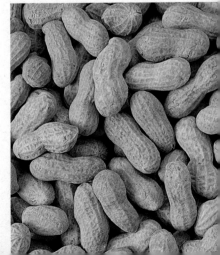

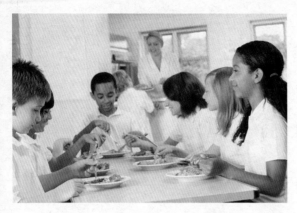

Because even peanut "dust" in the air can cause severe reactions in sensitive people, many school cafeterias no longer serve foods containing peanuts.

A minute amount of peanuts—for example peanut "dust" in the air caused by a nearby peanut muncher—may induce a severe reaction in sensitive individuals. As a result, many airlines have become peanut free, and many schools do not allow peanuts or peanut butter sandwiches in the classroom or cafeteria.

Peanuts are added to a large variety of processed foods, including dairy and nondairy frozen desserts (as a flavoring), cakes and cookies, marinades, salad dressings, sauces (especially Asian sauces), vegetarian burger patties, and a wide range of snack foods. Some individuals with peanut allergy have also shown reactions to sweet lupine seed flour, which may be added to some pastas, gluten-free baked goods, and other specialty food products.

Many manufacturing plants that process tree nut butters and seed butters also process peanut butters and other peanut products. Cross-contamination often is unavoidable. Consequently, individuals who are not allergic to tree nuts but are very sensitive to peanuts may not be able to eat prepared foods or other nut and seed butters that contain tree nuts.

Because food companies do not want to be responsible for an unforeseen peanut allergy reaction, many voluntarily place information about peanuts on food labels, such as the following: "Produced on shared equipment that processes products that contain peanuts," or "Produced at a facility that processes peanuts," or "May contain trace amounts of peanuts." This is a source of great comfort as well as great frustration to many peanut-allergy sufferers. It is important to note that because including allergy information on labels is voluntary, the lack of such a statement on a food product does not mean that it is free of peanut products. As the demand for peanut-free foods increases, we will be seeing more statements like "Produced in a peanut-free facility."

Peanut oil has generally been considered to be "safe," but like soy oil, its allergenicity appears to be related to the way the oil is processed. Cold-pressed peanut oils may contain peanut allergen, and the residual peanut proteins in it may become more allergenic with heating. Peanut

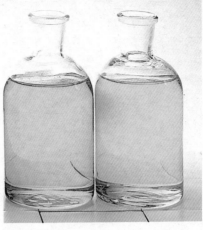

oil often is used to fry foods and is common in the preparation of many food and nonfood products, which can affect extremely sensitive individuals just through contact. Peanut oil may also be called arachis oil. Some skin lotions and hair products may contain peanut proteins. People who are sensitive to peanuts should select hypoallergenic cleansers and lotions whenever possible.

Living Without Peanuts: *Restaurants and traveling.* When dining outside of your peanut-free home, make it clear to the host or restaurant server and management that you have a peanut allergy that is severe. Ask if peanuts, peanut butter, and peanut oil are used and to what extent. Ask for recommendations that are peanut free. If you are at risk for anaphylaxis, always take your EpiPen with you in the case of unforeseen cross-contamination. Eateries that are most likely to use peanuts in many dishes include African, Chinese, Indonesian, Mexican, Thai, and Vietnamese restaurants.

Peanut oil may still contain residual proteins that will cause allergic reactions.

Food preparation without peanuts. Even though it is recommended that people who are hypersensitive to peanuts avoid *all* tree nuts (because of potential cross-contamination with peanuts), it is possible to find nuts that are "pure"—that is, that have never come into contact with peanuts via shared equipment or packaging facilities that also process peanuts. We contacted almond, pistachio, and other tree nut processors and discovered that some brands are peanut safe but don't necessarily say so on the label. We encourage you to call nut growers and manufacturers to find out which nuts and nut products are safe to buy in your area. You may also find ways to purchase nuts directly from the growers.

Being Well Nourished Without Peanuts Fortunately, the absence of peanuts from the diet poses no special risk of nutrient deficiencies. Peanuts are a good source of unsaturated fats, protein, vitamin E, and trace minerals. These nutrients also are abundant in tree nuts. If you can tolerate other nuts (and know of a reputable brand produced in a peanut-free facility), include them in your diet. If you wish to enjoy a peanut butter–like spread and you can tolerate tree nuts, try almond butter, cashew butter, soy nut butter, sunflower seed butter, and others. Be sure to purchase products processed in a peanut-free facility. You may be able to find other fresh nuts and seeds that are from a peanut-free facility; with these you can make your own nut and seed butters at home using a grinder, sturdy food processor, or juicer (several brands are suitable for making nut butters).

If you are sensitive to other nuts as well as peanuts and wish for a nutty spread, you have at least three options. One is I.M. Healthy brand soy nut butter (www.soynutbutter.com), which is made in a facility that is totally free of peanuts and tree nuts. The other is No Nuts brand Golden Pea Butter (www.peabutter.ca), made from special peas in a nut-free environment. SunButter (www.sunbutter.com) makes a sunflower seed butter in a factory that is completely free of peanuts and tree nuts.

Tree Nuts

Tree nut allergies are common and are potentially life threatening for some individuals; they often tend to persist for life. Tree nuts include almonds, brazil nuts, cashews, hazelnuts (filberts), macadamia nuts, pecans, pine nuts (pignolia nuts), pistachios, and walnuts. From an allergy perspective, the group labeled "tree nuts" does not include coconuts, nutmeg, peanuts, and water chestnuts. Almonds appear to be the least problematic of all common tree nuts. Some people suffer reactions from all of these nuts, and others from one or several. For those who experience anaphylaxis from exposure to one type of nut, all nuts should be avoided because all too often nuts are cross-contaminated with each other. (However, you might enjoy safe nuts directly from a grower or from a dedicated facility.) People allergic to peanuts often can eat tree nuts, and people allergic to tree nuts often can eat peanuts; some individuals are allergic to both.

People who react to one type of tree nut may or may not be sensitive to all types of tree nuts.

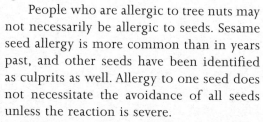

People who are allergic to tree nuts may not necessarily be allergic to seeds. Sesame seed allergy is more common than in years past, and other seeds have been identified as culprits as well. Allergy to one seed does not necessitate the avoidance of all seeds unless the reaction is severe.

Allergic reactions to nuts are most often caused by eating unlabelled foods, not checking food labels carefully, or consuming foods that contain hidden sources of nuts. The most common types of foods that cause allergic

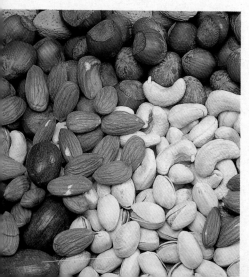

reactions attributable to nuts are candies, chocolates, cookies, granola bars, and ice creams. Symptoms of tree nut allergy range from tingling of the lips to anaphylactic shock. People sensitive to tree nuts may experience contact dermatitis (especially in the mouth); itching of the mouth, eyes, and ears; throat tightening; skin reactions; asthma; and intestinal discomfort.

Nuts may be found as a hidden, unlabelled part of a food because of accidental cross-contamination during manufacturing. Companies often label their products with the statement "may contain nuts" if they cannot guarantee that a food they are producing is free of nuts. This usually is because nuts are being used in the same machines for other foods. A company that makes similar foods—some that contain nuts and some that do not contain nuts—may have difficulty removing all traces of nut allergens when cleaning the machines between processing different items. This type of cross-contamination is most likely to occur with candies, cereals, chocolates, cookies, dried soups, ice creams, and nut butters. Chocolate and mint ice creams are most likely to contain undeclared nuts because leftover ice creams (from other production runs) can be added to these without changing the flavor. European chocolates are permitted to be made with leftover chocolate, which may contain nuts and may not be declared on the label.

Unpackaged foods, such as those in a cookie jar or tin, may contain traces of nuts from nut-containing cookies that were previously stored in the container. Bulk foods, buffet meals, and potluck dishes may also be dangerous because of cross-contamination. Cross-contamination can occur during food preparation when a cutting board or knife is used to chop nuts as well as other foods. It can also happen when the same oil is used to fry different foods, the same batter is used for different foods that are dipped into it, or the same frying utensils are used for different foods without being washed carefully between uses. Other possible sources of cross-contamination are coffee grinders (when nut-flavored coffees have been ground in them), muffin tins (when nut-containing batter is baked in them and the muffin tins are not properly cleaned), ice-cream scoops (when used for different flavors of ice

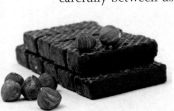

Candy and cookies can often be sources of cross-contamination.

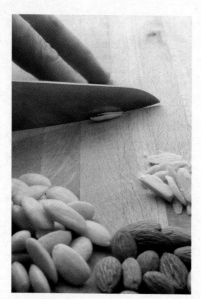

cream, including those that contain nuts), and knives (when used to cut a nut-containing dessert and then another dessert).

Allergic reactions can also be caused by vending machines that contain different foods at various times. If a vending machine previously contained nuts or nut-containing foods, other items in the machine may become contaminated with traces of nuts.

Safflower and canola oil do not need to be avoided unless someone is specifically allergic to them. It is believed that most tree nut oils probably contain enough allergenic protein to cause allergic reactions. "Cold-pressed" nut oils (those that are extruded or expressed without the use of chemicals and/or heat) are generally not safe for people who have nut-allergies.

Cross-contamination can happen when cutting boards, muffin tins, or ice cream scoops are used for nuts as well as other foods.

Living Without Tree Nuts: *Restaurants and traveling.* Once you are aware of the myriad ways that nuts can sneak their way into your diet, you should be able to dine outside your home without a high risk of exposure. Always ask your host or your restaurant server, as well as the restaurant manager, what options are available, and voice your concerns regarding your food allergies. Depending upon the severity of your reaction, you may need to avoid restaurants that use nuts as ingredients in their dishes.

Food preparation without tree nuts. Unless you are sensitive to all nuts, seeds, and soy, you can get creative in the kitchen with your cooking and baking. Try swapping a seed butter (such as tahini or sunflower butter) or soy nut butter for a tree nut butter in baked goods or sauces. Snack on roasted soybeans for a nutty crunch.

Being Well Nourished Without Tree Nuts Tree nuts provide protein, unsaturated fats, vitamin E, and the minerals calcium (in almonds), selenium (in brazil nuts), and zinc (especially in cashews). If you cannot tolerate any tree nuts at all, be sure to include a regular source of unsaturated fat in your diet, such as avocados, olives, and suitable vegetable oils. Seeds are a highly nutritious alternative for those who can tolerate them. Legumes (such as beans, peanuts, and soy) contain nutrients similar to those in nuts and are suitable substitutes in many main dishes.

Corn

Corn, which is often thought of as a vegetable, is actually a versatile grain. In addition to its widespread use in breakfast cereals, corn chips, corn tortillas, cornbread, grits, nachos, soups and chowders, side dishes, tacos, and, of course, corn on the cob, corn is the source of an inexpensive sweetener (corn syrup), thickener (cornstarch), and fat (corn oil) that are used extensively in the processed-food industry. People who are corn sensitive may suffer from intestinal distress, stuffy nose and sneezing, or hives after eating a food with corn in it. Corn allergy is relatively rare, but reactions may be severe among hypersensitive individuals. Nonallergic intolerance appears to be more prevalent than a true corn allergy.

Diets without corn are difficult to plan because corn and corn derivatives are used in many prepared foods and packaged products, mostly in the form of sweeteners or cornstarch. While it is easy to avoid obvious uses of corn in foods where corn is the featured ingredient (as with corn chips, corn tortillas, cornflakes, and popcorn), numerous processed foods contain corn derivatives that are more difficult to spot. Many packaged cereals and beverages are sweetened with corn syrup, and countless other pantry staples, such as baked beans, canned soups, and spaghetti sauce, contain corn oil, corn sweetener, or cornstarch.

Commercial food producers often make caramel flavoring with corn syrup instead of cane or beet sugar. Corn is used in maple, nut, and root beer flavorings for ice creams, ices, confections, and baked goods. Many fruit drinks and soft drinks contain corn syrup in their flavorings. Grits, hominy, maize, and polenta are also made with corn. Marshmallows are dusted with cornstarch to keep them from sticking together, and cornstarch is added to most brands of confectioner's sugar and baking powder to keep them from caking or clumping.

Corn may or may not be in food starch, modified food starch, vegetable gum, or vegetable starch. Contact the product manufacturer if these terms appear on an ingredient label to determine if they are corn derived (corn is not one of the allergens that must be stated on the food label). Distilled white vinegar, bleached white flour, and iodized table salt also may contain corn allergens.

Corn allergy is relatively rare, but reactions to corn may be severe.

39

Dextrin and maltodextrin, often made from cornstarch, are used in salad dressings, sauces, and ice creams as a thickening agent. Dextrose may be used in cookies, sports drinks, and crispy foods such as french fries, batter-fried foods, and potato puffs. Dextrose (also known as glucose or corn sugar) may be listed on labels as caramel, dextrin, dextrates, malt syrup, or maltodextrin.

Corn derivatives are used in a wide range of everyday products. These include general household goods, cosmetics, personal care products, and pharmaceuticals. Sometimes corn oil is used in emollient creams and toothpastes. Corn syrup often is used as a texturizer and carrying agent in cosmetics. Corn derivatives also may be found in adhesives, eating utensils made from recycled plastic, paper cups, paper plates, and plastic wrap. Other possible hidden sources of corn are aspirin, bath powders, laxatives, lozenges, medicinal capsules, ointments, suppositories, and vitamin supplements. Medications in liquid or tablet form may contain corn syrup or cornstarch.

Living Without Corn: *Restaurants and traveling.* Individuals who are sensitive to corn can still eat out, but it would be best to avoid Mexican restaurants, where corn ingredients are very common and cross-contamination may be inevitable. Asian restaurants may or may not be acceptable; ask the chefs what they use for thickening and sweetening sauces. Pizzas often are placed on a bed of cornmeal to prevent sticking, although you may be able to find a pizzeria that does not use cornmeal. You may have the most success at restaurants that take pride in using fresh ingredients and preparing everything to order; they may avoid processed ingredients that contain corn derivatives. Make your allergy clear to the restaurant host and management.

Food preparation without corn. Although ingredients like cornstarch and corn syrup are quite common in cooking and baking, acceptable substitutes are available. For recipes that call for cornstarch as a thickener, you can substitute arrowroot starch, kuzu starch, potato starch, or tapioca starch. Instead of corn syrup you

Corn ingredients are very common in Mexican restaurants, as well as some Asian restaurants

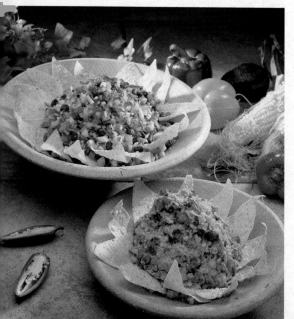

can use agave nectar, brown rice syrup, concentrated fruit juice, golden syrup (made from sugarcane), maple syrup, or molasses. (Note that these may affect the flavor, texture, and color of your finished product). Check out the sweeteners at your natural food store or gourmet market for corn-free options.

You don't need to give up snack foods that are typically corn based. Next time you watch a movie at home, try popped rice (available online and at many gourmet food stores), rice crisps, baked potato chips, vegetable chips, or even soy chips. Roll up your favorite fillings in a flour tortilla instead of a corn tortilla.

Being Well Nourished Without Corn Avoiding corn is not typically a cause for concern, nutritionally speaking. Multiple grain allergies, however, may be problematic. In that case, it is important to focus on whole foods that you are able to tolerate. Starchy vegetables, such as beets, parsnips, potatoes, radishes, sweet potatoes, turnips, and yams, are particularly well tolerated. These veggies provide a nutritious source of complex carbohydrates for grain-sensitive people. You can also try lesser known but equally tasty starchy vegetables such as cassava, Jerusalem artichokes, rutabaga, and taro.

Wheat

True wheat allergy is relatively uncommon. It is thought to affect fewer than 1 percent of infants, most of whom outgrow the allergy by the age of three, and it affects far fewer adults. However, self-reported sensitivity to wheat is becoming more common. Though the reason for the latter condition is not well understood, it appears that some people who are not actually allergic to wheat find that they feel better when they eliminate or cut down on wheat.

Like any food allergy, a wheat allergy may manifest as a respiratory reaction (such as wheezing), a skin response, or gastrointestinal distress. People who are severely sensitive to wheat may have reactions when their skin comes into contact with a wheat-containing food, when they breathe in wheat flour dust at a bakery ("baker's asthma," for example, is a respiratory allergy to inhaled flour), or inhale the allergen while harvesting wheat. Anaphylaxis to wheat is rare but does exist among some

True wheat allergy is uncommon, but self-reported wheat sensitivity appears to be increasing.

people. For people with a tendency to have this severe reaction, anaphylaxis may be induced by exercise.

Although you can be tested for wheat allergy at your allergist's office, the test results might not paint an accurate picture. Studies show that many people who test positive for a wheat allergy can eat wheat with no evidence of allergy symptoms. Conversely, people who exhibit obvious symptoms of allergy after consuming wheat may test negative for a wheat allergy. The best way to determine whether you are sensitive to wheat is to perform a careful elimination diet, followed by a food challenge (see page 18). During the elimination phase of the diet, it is important to avoid all possible sources of wheat.

Never assume that a product is wheat free simply because it appears to be so at first glance. For example, wheat proteins are common in seasoning mixtures and some food additives, the sources of which may not be identified on a food label (although, by law, they are required to be). Unless the product label specifically states "wheat free" and there are no ambiguous ingredients, it is possible that there are traces of wheat in the product. You might find that you can tolerate such tiny amounts of wheat; carefully monitoring of your intake, along with observing any symptoms you experience, will help you determine how much wheat, if any, your body can handle without consequence. Fortunately, there is an enormous market for wheat-free products, so your prospects for enjoying a wheat-free life are excellent and improving all the time.

Living Without Wheat: *Restaurants and traveling.* Probably the most challenging aspect of following a wheat-free diet is dining outside your home. Our kitchens are safe havens where we know exactly how our food is prepared. When we eat at the home of a friend or relative, or at a restaurant, we must be especially careful. If you are very sensitive to wheat, it's best to avoid places that make their own bread or pasta because wheat flour can contaminate foods that are otherwise wheat free. Talk to the manager of the restaurant you're visiting and be specific about what you can and cannot eat. Your best option may be to order basic, straightforward foods, such as salads, grilled or steamed vegetables, rice, and fresh fruit. Because condiments, salad dressings, and sauces are common sources of "hidden" wheat, it's wise to take along your own salad dressing, sauce, or wheat-free seasonings. Many natural-food and vegetarian restaurants now offer wheat-free delicacies like quinoa salad, rice pilaf, and millet-bean burgers. (See restaurant choices at www.happycow.net.) As awareness of wheat sensitivity grows, so will our food selections, both inside and outside of our homes.

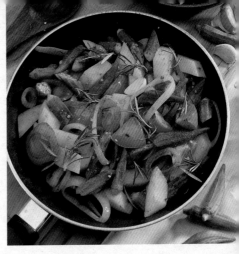

Food preparation without wheat. Thanks to the myriad wheat-free products and recipes available, you can eat almost "normally"— that is, much like a person who eats wheat does! For breakfast you might enjoy a wheat-free cereal topped with fortified rice milk or soymilk and fresh fruit. For lunch, how about a hearty bean soup with some wheat-free bread or rice crackers. For supper, enjoy wheat-free noodles or rice with sautéed vegetables in a succulent sauce, accompanied by a crisp garden salad. Even though you cannot have wheat, your meal and snack options are extensive.

A good option when eating out is ordering basic foods, such as grilled or steamed vegetables.

Being Well Nourished Without Wheat Wheat provides B vitamins (including folic acid and riboflavin), carbohydrates (including fiber, if the whole grain is left intact), iron, magnesium, zinc, and protein. Fortunately, alternative grains provide similar and often superior nutritional quality—quinoa and amaranth are two excellent examples. Include plenty of wheat-free grains: amaranth, buckwheat, millet, and quinoa. Enjoy wheat-free versions of bagels, breads, pizza, and sweets (but don't become overly dependent on them; too many of these products can displace more nutritious foods in the diet). Consume plenty of fresh fruits, vegetables, and legumes (beans, lentils, and peas).

Other Food Culprits

There are many other foods to which we may develop sensitivities. In this section we briefly discuss other triggers for allergic reactions.

Fish and Shellfish Fish, crustaceans (such as crab, crayfish, lobster, and shrimp), and mollusks (such as clams, mussels, oysters, and scallops) are among the most potent allergens. People who have a potentially life-threatening anaphylactic reaction are advised to avoid all fish because of the proteins they contain known as parvalbumins. Those who are sensitive to one crustacean are likely to be sensitive to all types of crustaceans; the same is true for mollusks.

If you are allergic to fish, note that worcestershire sauce contains anchovies and may be found in Caesar salad dressing, caponata relish, cocktails, and pasta sauce. Anchovies may also be found on pizzas.

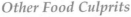

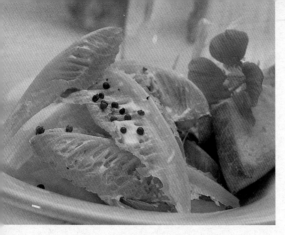

Anchovies are usually an ingredient in the worcestershire sauce found in Caesar salads and some Asian foods.

Asian food may contain oyster sauce or worcestershire sauce. Miso soup may contain fish extract, and Thai curries may contain fish sauce. Avoid french fries from restaurants that use the same oil for fries and fish. Shampoos, conditioners, and other skin care products may contain fish oils. In fish and seafood restaurants there is a risk of cross-contamination from utensils and cooking surfaces in the food-preparation areas. Fish protein can become airborne; some individuals have had reactions from just walking through a fish market.

Fish is touted as an important source of omega-3 fatty acids, but flaxseeds, hempseeds, soy foods, and walnuts are also good sources. Several plant-based brands of omega-3 capsules can be found in the resource section on page 63.

Sesame Seeds and Other Seeds Sesame seeds may be a cause of allergic reactions, typically around the mouth or in the digestive or respiratory systems. They may be anaphylactic for some individuals. Some find that all seeds pose problems; for others, one type of seed is problematic but others cause no reaction. Seeds that are an ingredient in other foods (for example, in baked goods, breads, or energy bars) are chia, cottonseed, flax, hemp, melon, pomegranate, psyllium, pumpkin, sesame, and sunflower. Seeds that are used as seasonings include celery, fennel, mustard (black, yellow, and white), poppy, and others. Flaxseed oil and sesame oil may contain traces of protein allergens.

Sesame seeds are present in tahini (sesame paste), hummus, and halva. They are a common ingredient in bagels, breadsticks, crackers, falafel, and pretzels. Sesame seed oils are present in the herbal beverage Aqua Libra and are often an ingredient in Chinese stir-fries. The antioxidant vitamin E, also known as a tocopherol, is sometimes extracted from seeds, including sesame seeds.

Latex, Banana, Kiwifruit, Avocado, and Chestnut Though this may seem an odd grouping, remember that rubber comes from a tree. Those who are allergic to latex rubber (found in baby-bottle nipples, balloons, condoms, dental dams, or gloves) are sometimes allergic to certain foods, most notably avocados, bananas, or chestnuts, and sometimes kiwifruit, mangoes, peaches, and certain other foods. Not everyone with a latex allergy will react to the whole list; at least twelve potentially allergenic proteins can be involved. Latex reaction can be anaphylactic.

Cross Reactivity among Plant Families Prior to the 1980s, the popular assumption was that a person allergic to the edible part of one plant was allergic to other plants within the same botanical family or would become so if foods from the other plants were ingested. It has since been learned that we react to specific allergenic proteins in a particular food. A particular food often contains several proteins that may be antigens, and we may react to one, or several, but not all of those antigens. Plant A may contain one protein that is also present in plant B, whereas a second allergenic protein may be found in plants A and C but not in B. There is no scientific reason to assume that we are allergic to foods in related botanical families, and there is no need to excessively restrict foods. Our response patterns are unique and are not necessarily identical to those of other people who react to one of the same foods that we do.

Conclusion

Your discovery of food allergies may be the dawn of a new way of eating that, over time, will reveal benefits far beyond what you expect. Although some items are off the menu now, your food horizons may just be opening up. Your allergic reactions can inspire you to adopt simple habits that will eventually prove highly beneficial. In spite of your diet being somewhat different from those around you, yours can be wonderfully healthful and delicious and provide every nutrient you require. In other words, your food allergies may turn out to be a blessing.

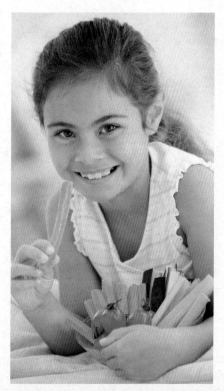

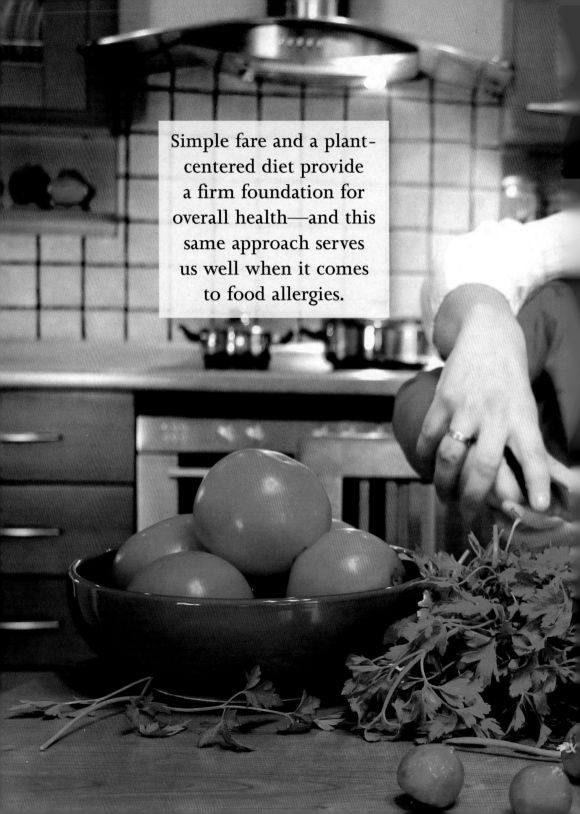

Simple fare and a plant-centered diet provide a firm foundation for overall health—and this same approach serves us well when it comes to food allergies.

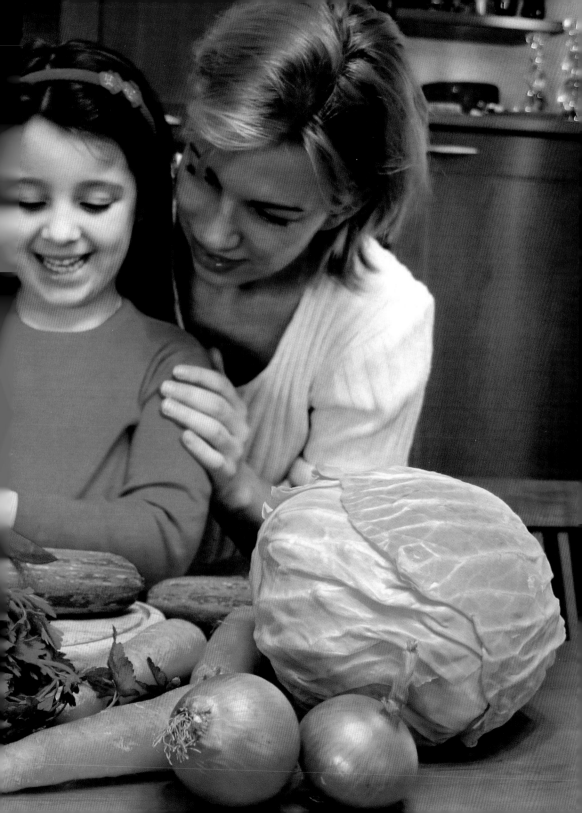

Creamy Carrot Bisque with Exotic Spices

Although there are no dairy products in this exotically flavored soup, the texture is incredibly creamy. In addition to the beta-carotene, which gives the soup its vivid color, it is rich in essential though less well-known minerals: chromium, copper, magnesium, manganese, molybdenum, phosphorus, and potassium.

2 tablespoons (30 ml) olive oil

1 large onion, coarsely chopped

1 pound (454 g) carrots, trimmed, scraped, and sliced

1 large potato, peeled and coarsely chopped

½ teaspoon (2 ml) ground cardamom

½ teaspoon (2 ml) ground cinnamon

¼ teaspoon (1 ml) ground ginger

¼ teaspoon (1 ml) ground nutmeg

Salt and cayenne

7 cups (1.75 L) hot vegetable stock or water

Heat the oil in a large soup pot. Add the onion and sauté for 5 minutes. Add the carrots and potato and stir until coated with the oil. Add the cardamom, cinnamon, ginger, nutmeg and salt, and cayenne to taste and sauté for 10 minutes. Pour in the hot stock or water and bring to a boil. Reduce the heat, cover, and simmer until the vegetables are very tender, about 30 minutes. Purée in batches in a blender until smooth. Serve hot.

Yields about 7 cups (1.75 L)

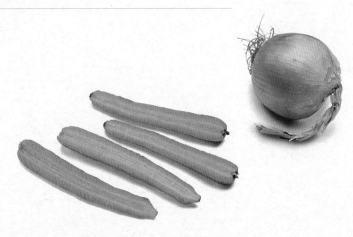

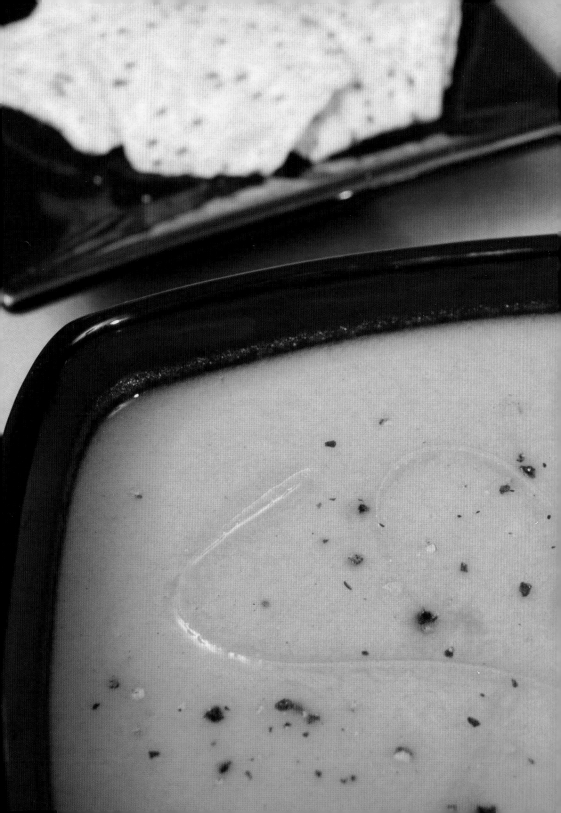

Confetti Coleslaw

Fresh flavors and bright colors combine to make this coleslaw stand out from the ordinary. It's a delicious accompaniment to spicy chili or any bean dish or soup, and it's always a potluck favorite.

2 cups (500 ml) thinly sliced or shredded red cabbage

½ cup (125 ml) thinly sliced or shredded green cabbage

1 large carrot, shredded

1 red or yellow bell pepper, finely diced

½ small red onion, thinly sliced

3 tablespoons (45 ml) extra-virgin olive oil

2 tablespoons (30 ml) red or white wine vinegar

1 teaspoon (5 ml) sugar or other sweetener of your choice

½ teaspoon (2 ml) prepared yellow mustard

Salt and pepper

Combine the cabbage, carrot, pepper, and onion in a large bowl and toss well. Whisk together the remaining ingredients and pour over the vegetables. Toss to thoroughly combine. Chill for at least 1 hour before serving.

Yields about 4 cups (1 L)

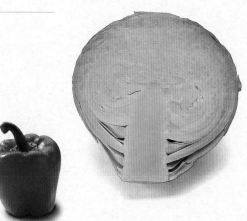

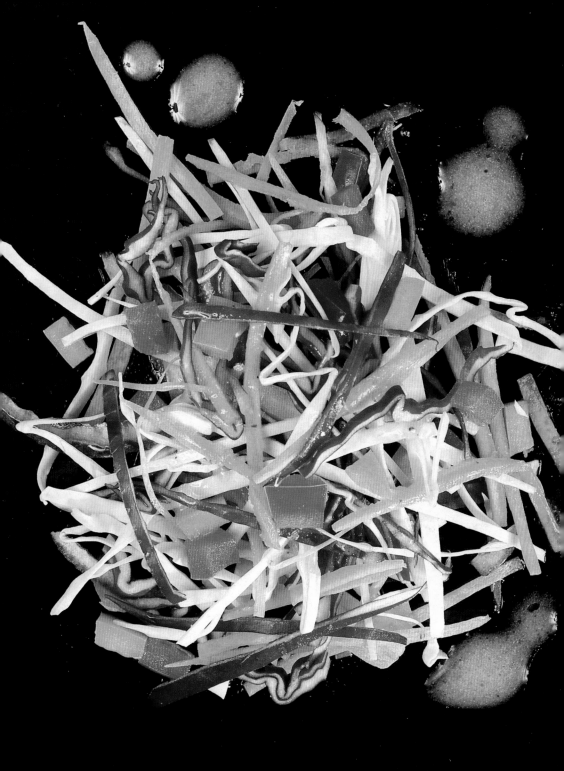

Ruby Wild Rice Salad

This salad fits the bill for holiday gatherings and other special occasions, as well as everyday feasts. It is made with dried cranberries, which look like glistening rubies. Radishes and seeds add crunch.

4 cups (1000 ml) cooked wild rice (about 1¾ cups/ 435 ml dry)

1¼ cups (310 ml) diced daikon (Japanese radish) or other radishes

1 cup (250 ml) sunflower or pumpkin seeds, lightly pan toasted

1 cup (250 ml) sweetened dried cranberries

1 orange, yellow, or red bell pepper, diced

½ cup (125 ml) sliced scallions

⅓ cup (85 ml) orange juice

2 tablespoons (30 ml) balsamic vinegar

2 tablespoons (30 ml) extra-virgin olive oil

1 teaspoon (5 ml) Dijon mustard

Salt and pepper

Combine the cooked wild rice, daikon, seeds, cranberries, bell pepper, and scallions in a large bowl. Toss to mix. In a separate small bowl, whisk together the orange juice, vinegar, oil, and mustard until well combined. Pour over the salad and toss gently until evenly distributed. Season with salt and pepper to taste. Chill or serve at once.

Yields about 8½ cups (2.125 L)

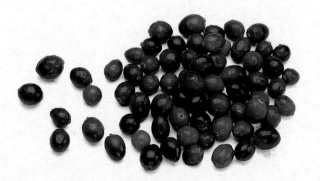

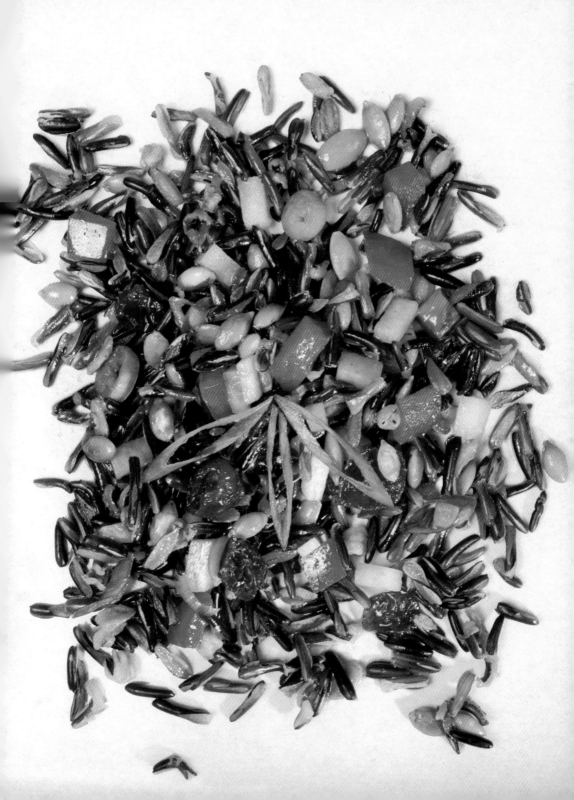

Black Bean Tostadas

Enjoy this south-of-the-border specialty with plenty of your favorite toppings.

1¾ cups (435 ml) drained cooked black beans or one (15-ounce/425-g) can

1 tablespoon (15 ml) balsamic vinegar or fresh lime juice

2 teaspoons (10 ml) chili powder

1 teaspoon (5 ml) garlic powder

½ teaspoon (2 ml) ground cumin

½ teaspoon (2 ml) dried oregano

Salt

Tabasco

8 corn tortillas

½ cup (125 ml) finely chopped onions

Toppings (select one or more):

1–2 cups (250–500 ml) shredded romaine or leaf lettuce

2 ripe tomatoes, chopped

1 small avocado, cut into chunks

½ cup (125 ml) shredded carrot

½ cup (125 ml) prepared salsa

½ cup (125 ml) sliced black olives

¼ cup (60 ml) finely chopped red onions

Coarsely chop the beans by hand or by pulsing them briefly in a food processor. Combine the chopped beans, vinegar, chili powder, garlic powder, cumin, oregano, and add salt and Tabasco to taste. Toss until thoroughly combined.

Warm the tortillas one by one in a dry skillet, then stack them in a clean towel to keep them warm. Heat the oil in the skillet. When hot, add the onions and sauté until tender, about 10–15 minutes. Add the bean mixture to the skillet and sauté until warmed through and just starting to brown, about 5 minutes. Spoon an equal portion of the bean mixture onto each of the reserved tortillas. Add your favorite toppings, or place bowls of several different toppings on the table. To eat, gently fold the tortillas, and pick them up with your hands.

Yields 4–8 servings
(1 or 2 tostadas per person)

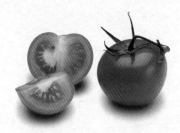

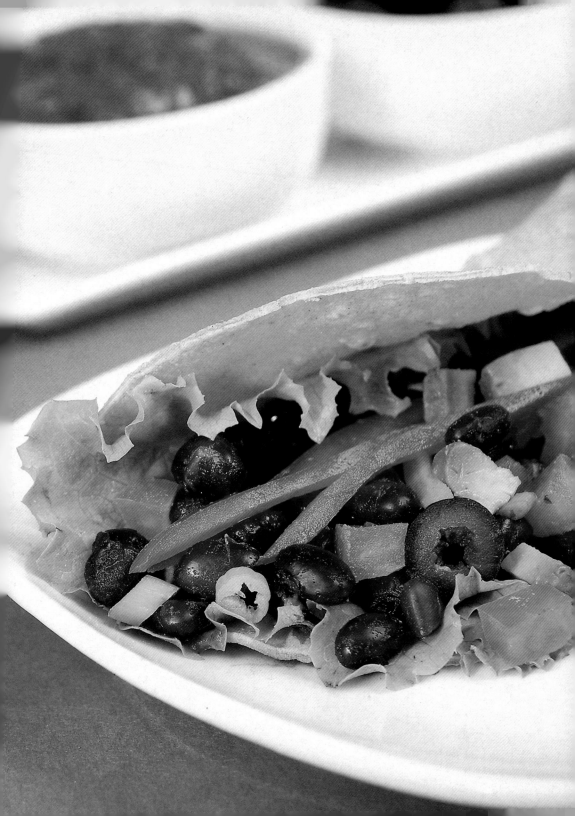

Hearty Bean Stew

Enjoy old-fashioned beef-stew flavor with a new twist—beans instead of beef!

4 cups (1 L) diced potatoes (thin-skinned or peeled)

4 large carrots, sliced in half lengthwise and cut into 1-inch (2.5 cm) chunks

2 cups (500 ml) vegetable broth or water

2 stalks celery, finely chopped

2 bay leaves

1 tablespoon (15 ml) extra-virgin olive oil

1 cup (250 ml) chopped onions

2 cups (500 ml) sliced mushrooms

3 tablespoons (45 ml) rice flour

2 tablespoons (30 ml) sesame tahini or other seed butter

3 tablespoons (45 ml) chickpea miso

½ cup (125 ml) water

2 cups drained (500 ml) cooked beans of choice or 1 (15- or 16-ounce/ 425- to 450-g) can

Salt and pepper

Yields 4 servings

Place the potatoes, carrots, broth, celery, and bay leaves in a large saucepan or pot. Bring to a boil, reduce the heat to medium, cover, and simmer, stirring occasionally, until the vegetables are tender, about 20 minutes.

Meanwhile, place the oil in a large skillet over medium-high heat. Add the onions and sauté for 8 minutes or until almost tender. Add the mushrooms and continue to sauté until tender, about 4–6 minutes longer.

Remove the skillet from the heat and stir in the flour. Mix well. Then stir in the seed butter and mix well. Dissolve the miso in the water, then gradually stir it into the skillet mixture, mixing vigorously until the sauce is smooth. Stir this mixture into the hot cooked vegetables and their liquid and mix well.

Stir in the cooked beans and bring to a boil, stirring almost constantly. Reduce the heat to medium and continue to stir and simmer the stew just until the sauce thickens, about 3–5 minutes. Remove the bay leaves and season with salt and pepper. Ladle into bowls and serve hot.

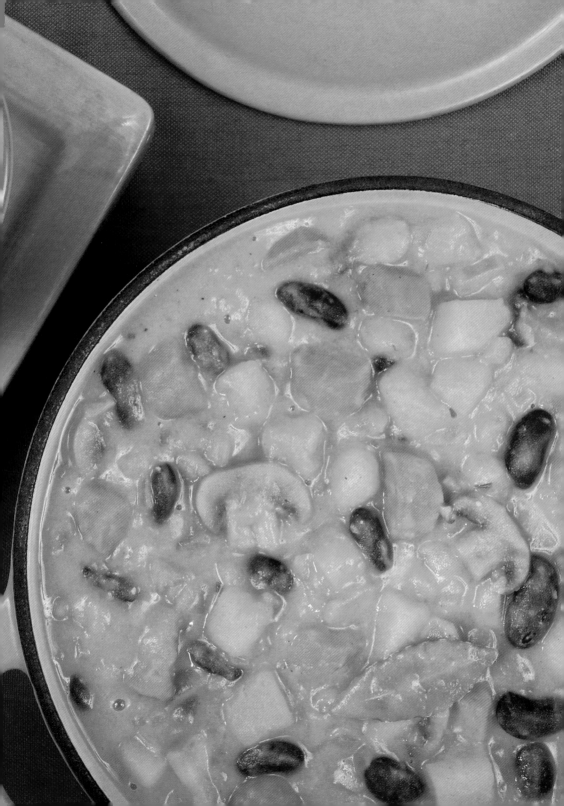

Moroccan Millet

This pilaf is great as a one-dish meal or served with a fresh green salad.

2 tablespoons (30 ml) coconut or olive oil or organic canola or safflower oil

1 large red bell pepper, sliced into strips

1 large green bell pepper, sliced into strips

1 large onion, sliced into half-moons

2 tablespoons (30 ml) crushed garlic

2 teaspoons (10 ml) paprika

½ teaspoon (2 ml) salt

1 teaspoon (5 ml) ground cumin

½ teaspoon (2 ml) ground cinnamon

¼ teaspoon (1 ml) turmeric

¼ teaspoon (1 ml) ground ginger

⅛ teaspoon cayenne (1 pinch)

1½ cups (375 ml) millet

3 cups (750 ml) vegetable stock

1¾ cups (435 ml) drained cooked chickpeas or 1 (15-ounce/425-g) can

¼ cup (60 ml) raisins or chopped dates

¼ cup (60 ml) sunflower seeds, pumpkin seeds, or pine nuts (optional)

Salt and pepper

Yields about 6 servings

Preheat the oven to 450°F (230°C). Place 1 tablespoon (15 ml) of the oil in a large roasting pan. Add the peppers, onion, garlic, paprika, and salt. Toss until everything is evenly coated with the oil and well combined. Place in the oven to roast for 20 minutes, stirring 2 or 3 times during the cooking cycle. Remove the vegetables from the oven and allow them to cool until safe to handle; then chop them coarsely.

Meanwhile, heat the remaining tablespoon (15 ml) of oil in a large saucepan. Add the cumin, cinnamon, turmeric, ginger, and cayenne. Stir over medium-high heat until the spices are uniform in color and well combined, about 30 seconds. Add the millet and stir quickly to coat, about 1 minute. Immediately pour in the vegetable stock and bring to a boil. Reduce the heat, cover, and cook the millet until all the liquid is absorbed, about 20 minutes.

Place the millet in a large bowl and fluff with a fork. Add the roasted vegetables, chickpeas, raisins, and optional seeds. Season with salt and pepper to taste. Toss gently and serve.

Du Toit G, Katz Y, Sasieni P, Mesher D, et al. Early consumption of peanuts in infancy is associated with a low prevalence of peanut allergy. *J Allergy Clin Immunol*. 2008 Nov;122(5):984–91.

Greer FR, Sicherer SH, Burks AW; American Academy of Pediatrics Committee on Nutrition; American Academy of Pediatrics Section on Allergy and Immunology. Effects of early nutritional interventions on the development of atopic disease in infants and children: the role of maternal dietary restriction, breast-feeding, timing of introduction of complementary foods, and hydro-lyzed formulas. *Pediatrics*. 2008 Jan;121(1):183–91.

Institute of Medicine (IOM). *Dietary Reference Intakes for Energy, Carbohydrates, Fiber, Fat, Protein and Amino Acids (Macronutrients)*, Washington, DC: National Acade-mies Press; 2002. Available at www.nap.educatalog.php?record_id=10490. Accessed March 2010.

Joneja JV. *Dealing with Food Aller-gies: a practical guide to detecting culprit foods and eating a healthy, enjoyable diet*. Bull Publishing, Colorado, 2003.

Joneja JV. *Dealing with Food Aller-gies in Babies and Children*. Bull Publishing, Colorado, 2007.

WHO, Consultation FAO. Diet, nutrition and the prevention of chronic diseases. *WHO Technical Report Series 916*. Geneve: WHO. 2003;916.

Wood RA. The natural history of food allergy. *Pediatrics*. 2003;111 (6):1631–7.

For further nutrition information, practical tips, plus a wealth of outstanding recipes that are free of all of the top allergens, see *Food Allergy Survival Guide* by Vesanto Melina, Jo Stepaniak, and Dina Aronson.

Sources for plant-based omega-3 fatty acids

Pangea
www.veganstore.com
800-340-1200

Vegan Essentials
www.veganessentials.com
866-88-VEGAN

Contact these suppliers for the following brands:
O-Mega-Zen3
Deva Omega-3 DHA
Spectrum Vegetarian DHA
V-Pure by Water4Life
Pure One

Published by **Books Alive**
PO Box 99
Summertown, TN 38483
931-964-3571
888-260-8458

Book Design:
    Cynthia Holzapfel
    Warren Jefferson
Art Direction:
    Warren Jefferson
Recipe Development:
    Jo Stepaniak
    Vesanto Melina
    Dina Aronson
Recipe Photography:
    Warren Jefferson
Food Styling:
    Barbara Jefferson
Photo Editing:
    Cynthia Holzapfel
Editing:
    Jo Stepaniak

Library of Congress Cataloging-in-Publication Data
Stepaniak, Joanne,
  Food allergies : health and healing / Jo Stepaniak, Vesanto Melina, and Dina Aronson.
    p. cm.
  Includes bibliographical references and index.
  ISBN 978-1-55312-046-9 (alk. paper)
  1. Food allergy--Popular works. 2. Food allergy--Diet therapy--Popular works. I. Melina, Vesanto, 1942- II. Aronson, Dina L. III. Title.
  RC596.S74 2010
  616.97'50654--dc22   2010016177

ISBN 978-1-55312-046-9
Printed in Hong Kong

Alive Natural Health Guides

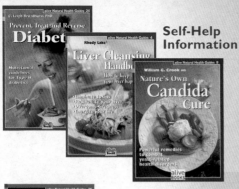

Self-Help Information

Prevent, Treat and Reverse
Diabet

Rhody Lake
Liver Cleansing
Handb

William G. Crook MD
Nature's Own
Candida Cure

Powerful remedies
to combat
yeast-related
health disorders

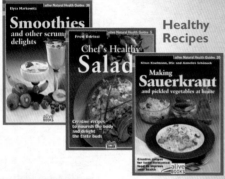

Healthy Recipes

Elysa Markowitz
Smoothies
and other scrum
delights

Fred Edrissi
Chef's Healthy
Salad

Klaus Kaufmann, DSc and Annelies Schöneck
Making
Sauerkraut
and pickled vegetables at home

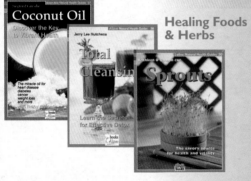

Healing Foods & Herbs

Coconut Oil
Discover the Key
to Vibrant Health

Jerry Lee Hutchens
Total Cleansin

Kathleen O'Bannon CNC
Sprouts

The savory source
for health and vitality

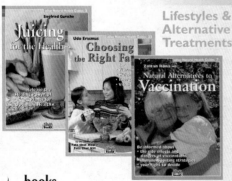

Lifestyles & Alternative Treatments

Siegfried Gursche
Juicing
for the Health

Udo Erasmus
Choosing
the Right Fa

Zoltan Rona MD
Natural Alternatives to
Vaccination

Be informed about
• the side effects and
dangers of vaccination
• immune-boosting strategies
• your right to decide

About the authors . . . .

Jo Stepaniak is author of over a dozen books (including *The Ultimate Uncheese Cookbook* and *Raising Vegetarian Children*) and hundreds of articles on vegetarian cuisine and compassionate living.

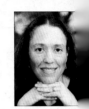

Vesanto Melina is a registered dietitian, has taught nutrition at Bastyr University in Seattle, Washington, and is coauthor of the *American Dietetic Association and Dietitians of Canada's Position on Vegetarian Diets (2003)* and *Manual of Clinical Dietetics, 6th ed., 2000.*

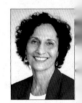

Dina Aronson has written for the *Journal of the American Dietetic Association* and *Today's Dietitian*, and is co-author of *Minerals from Plant Foods: Strategies for Maximizing Nutrition.*

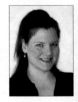

About this series . . . .

The ***Alive Natural Health Guides*** is the first series of its kind in North America. Each book focuses on a specific natural health related topic and explains how you can improve your health and lifestyle through diet and natural healing methods.

**books
Alive**
Summertown
Tennessee

1-800-695-2241   www.healthy-eating.com